Guided Meditation

Experience Blissful Balance With the Power of Chakra Healing

(Unlock the Power of Chakra Awakening and Get More Deep Sleep Through Meditation)

Paul Crawford

Published By **Percy Clint**

Paul Crawford

All Rights Reserved

Guided Meditation: Experience Blissful Balance With the Power of Chakra Healing (Unlock the Power of Chakra Awakening and Get More Deep Sleep Through Meditation)

ISBN 978-1-7772636-3-8

No part of this guidebook shall be reproduced in any form without permission in writing from the publisher except in the case of brief quotations embodied in critical articles or reviews.

Legal & Disclaimer

The information contained in this book is not designed to replace or take the place of any form of medicine or professional medical advice. The information in this book has been provided for educational & entertainment purposes only.

The information contained in this book has been compiled from sources deemed reliable, and it is accurate to the best of the Author's knowledge; however, the Author cannot guarantee its accuracy and validity and cannot be held liable for any errors or omissions. Changes are periodically made to this book. You must consult your doctor or get professional medical advice before using any of the suggested remedies, techniques, or information in this book.

Upon using the information contained in this book, you agree to hold harmless the Author from and against any damages, costs, and expenses, including any legal fees potentially resulting from the application of any of the information provided by this guide. This disclaimer applies to any damages or injury caused by the use and application, whether directly or indirectly, of any advice or information presented, whether for breach of contract, tort, negligence, personal injury, criminal intent, or under any other cause of action.

You agree to accept all risks of using the information presented inside this book. You need to consult a professional medical practitioner in order to ensure you are both able and healthy enough to participate in this program.

Table Of Contents

Chapter 1: Tarot Meditation Basics 1

Chapter 2: The Number One Symbols Of The Tarot Playing Cards 15

Chapter 3: The Meaning of the Minor Arcana 26

Chapter 4: Preparation and Attunement to Meditation 41

Chapter 5: Visualization Techniques in the Tarot Meditation Process 50

Chapter 6: The Importance of Colors and Symbols in Meditation 63

Chapter 7: The Role of Dreams in Tarot Meditation 72

Chapter 8: Tarot Meditation in Exquisite Areas of Life 81

Chapter 9: The Importance of Ritual in Tarot Meditation 90

Chapter 10: Developing Intuition through Tarot Meditation 100

Chapter 11: What Exactly Is Meditation? 106

Chapter 12: What Takes Location While You Meditate? 114

Chapter 13: Learn the Art and Basic Techniques with These Pointers 139

Chapter 14: Mindfulness for Teens 150

Chapter 15: Understanding Stress 164

Chapter 16: Guided Meditation 170

Chapter 17: Designing Your Guided Meditation Sessions 176

Chapter 1: Tarot Meditation Basics

Welcome to Tarot Meditation for Beginners: Unlocking Intuitive Wisdom. In this manual we're able to find out the captivating worldwide of Tarot meditation together. Before we dive into the depths of this workout, it's far critical to apprehend the basics.

Tarot meditation is a effective manner to increase intuition, find out internal knowledge and sell non secular growth. However, in advance than embarking on this journey, it's far essential to construct a solid basis.

What is Tarot Meditation?

Tarot meditation combines the visible symbolism of tarot cards with the ideas of meditation. Tarot playing cards act like a reflect of the subconscious, allowing you to delve deeper into your very own psyche. The mixture of meditation and tarot opens a space for self-records and spiritual development.

Choosing and being concerned for the tarot deck

Before you begin tarot meditation, it's miles essential to select the right tarot deck for you. Take the time to check outstanding decks and enjoy which one appeals to you. The deck might be a reliable associate for your journey.

Introduction to smooth tarot card symbols

Tarot playing playing cards have many symbols and photos that hint at deeper meanings. Learn the primary symbols of tarot gambling cards, which encompass the factors hearth, water, air and earth. Understand how these symbols relate to your own spirituality.

Meaning of the Major Arcana

The Major Arcana shape the coronary heart of the Tarot deck. Each card represents a section of lifestyles or an important revel in. Immerse yourself within the mystical international of these playing playing cards and discover that they're the vital element for your inner know-how.

The that means of the Minor Arcana

The Minor Arcana deepens the message of the Major Arcana. They reflect normal evaluations and worrying situations. Understand the four Tarot suites - Cups, Wands, Swords and Pentacles - and their respective meanings.

Meaning of the 4 tarot suites

The tarot suites constitute awesome areas of lifestyles. The cup represents feelings, the employees represents strength and motion, the sword represents thoughts and communique, and the coin represents rely and finance. Learn a manner to apply these symbols in meditation.

Preparation and attunement to meditation

Learn a way to great put together for a Tarot meditation. Create a quiet location, light a candle and take a seat down outcomes. Immerse your self within the second and music in to the enjoy you're about to have.

Breathing for deep meditation

Breathing is a powerful manner to immerse yourself in meditation. Discover extremely good respiratory techniques to calm your mind and popularity at the tarot playing cards. Breathing creates a connection many of the outdoor global and the internal self.

Visualization strategies in Tarot meditation

Visualization is an critical problem of Tarot meditation. Learn the manner to convey the gambling cards' symbols to life and embody them into your imagination. This allows you to connect greater deeply with the messages the tarot conveys to you.

Conscious relaxation

Relaxation is the essential thing to a success tarot meditation. You will discover ways to consciously allow go in order to supply area to the inner guidance of the tarot playing gambling cards. Conscious rest opens the door to hidden insights.

Meditation with Tarot playing cards - a step-through-step guide

Finally, it's time for the actual Tarot meditation. You'll be guided thru a step-with the resource of-step meditation in that you pick out out out a tarot card and discover its message for your self. This practical manual will will will let you placed concept into exercise. The which means of colors and logos in meditation

The suits and logos of the tarot playing gambling playing cards have deep meanings. Dive into the psychology of colours and look at the manner they've an impact on your temper. Understand the symbolism within the back of the styles and comprise them into your very very personal interpretation.

Explore your intuition.

Tarot meditation promotes the development of instinct. Listen for your internal impulses and find out how your instinct can guide you.

Your intuition is a precious compass on the direction to self-know-how.

The Role of Dreams in Tarot Meditation

Dreams often reflect our innermost desires and fears. Learn the manner to include desires into your tarot meditation and discover the hidden factors of your unconscious. Dreams can be the critical issue to new insights.

Overcoming boundaries - recommendations for a fulfillment meditation

Obstacles may upward push up at the course of tarot meditation. This is probably restlessness of thoughts or doubts approximately your skills. Learn the way to turn out to be aware about and overcome the ones barriers to enjoy a fulfillment and appealing meditation.

Tarot meditations for particular regions of existence

Tarot meditations are various. Learn a manner to apply this meditation to first-rate areas of existence, which encompass relationships, career, and personal increase. Tarot playing gambling playing cards can be a reliable partner for a satisfying lifestyles.

Incorporate meditation into your each day lifestyles.

Regular Tarot meditation exercise has a transformative effect. You will discover methods to mix the insights and internal peace you benefit into your every day lifestyles. Tarot meditation as a consequence becomes a supply of perception and balance.

The significance of rituals in tarot meditation

Rituals create a deep connection to what we do. Learn a way to create a sacred and collaborative environment with the aid of manner of incorporating ritual into your Tarot meditation. Rituals anchor the exercising on your cognizance and deepen the revel in.

Dealing with feelings throughout meditation

Emotions are a natural a part of tarot meditation. Learn to deal with one among a type feelings, which includes delight, disappointment and marvel. Tarot gambling playing cards will will let you boom a aware method on your feelings.

Develop your instinct with Tarot meditation

Finally, we can check the lengthy-term consequences of tarot meditation. You will learn the manner your intuition deepens over time and the manner you can use those insights to live a satisfying and conscious life.

If you recognize the fundamentals of this Tarot meditation, you may lay the inspiration for a charming journey to yourself. In the subsequent chapters you could deepen individual components and practical carrying events. Take it slow with every step and enjoy the magic of tarot meditation. Your journey starts offevolved now.

Choosing and Care for a Tarot Deck

Now that we've located out the basics of tarot meditation, allow's circulate immediately to the following important step: selecting and keeping a tarot deck.

The significance of creating the proper choice

Choosing a tarot deck can be very crucial. Take the time to preserve precise decks on your arms and revel in which one connects collectively along side your intuition. Whether it is a rider-weight, tote, or present day deck, select one which appeals on your internal senses.

Senses and impressions

Close your eyes and enjoy what sensations and impressions the deck triggers in you. Pay interest to your instinct as you look through the playing cards. Your first impressions are often the guiding stars in your journey of self-discovery.

Caring in your tarot deck

Your tarot deck can be a dedicated partner to your religious adventure. Handle your tarot deck with care. Keep it in a completely unique region and create an energetically excellent surroundings. A fabric or container will help defend it from dust and horrible affects.

Cleaning the tarot deck

Energy accumulates inside the gambling cards. Clean the deck often to cast off vintage strength. You can burn incense with sage or cleaning herbs. Imagine the horrible strength disappearing and being changed with the aid of natural, super vibrations.

Reload the tarot deck.

Once the cleaning is whole, recharge your tarot deck. Place it inside the moderate of the full moon or within the solar. Imagine that the gambling playing cards are being charged with new energy. This system strengthens the connection among you and the cards.

Connection with the cardboard hobby

Learn the manner to create a deeper connection with the tarot deck. Sit quietly, preserve the deck in your palms and near your eyes. Feel the power flowing amongst you and the gambling cards. This connection will deepen through the years and offer you with a wealthy supply of concept.

Choose the right deck for you.

There are infinite tarot decks within the marketplace. Some are conventional, a few present day and a few revolutionary. Find a deck that fits your person and spiritual route. It does not have to be the maximum well-known one, however one that speaks to your soul.

The function of instinct within the choice technique

Intuition performs an crucial feature at the equal time as deciding on a tarot deck. Imagine your self interacting with the playing cards. Feel whether the gambling gambling cards can provide you with answers or insights. Trust your instinct. Your instinct will guide you to the right deck for you.

Tarot decks for beginners

Rider-Waite and one of a kind traditional decks are often endorsed if you are new to the world of tarot. They are correct for beginners because of the truth the symbols are clean and smooth to interpret. Later, while you experience prepared, you can circulate on to more complicated decks.

Taking care of the tarot deck as a ritual

Taking care of your tarot deck can be a precious ritual. Sit down frequently to smooth and recharge your playing cards. Use this time to consciousness to your religious journey. Rituals create a deeper connection and deepen your courting with the playing cards.

The significance of the primary draw

Once you've got were given received your new deck of playing cards, the number one draw is a completely unique enjoy. Look for fashionable messages and clues for your religious journey. The first draw units the muse for the relationship among you and the deck.

The connection amongst you and the cards

By putting in a deep reference to the Tarot deck, the Tarot deck turns into a living tool of intuition. The playing cards are not only a tool, they're additionally a reflected photograph of your internal information. Explore precise tarot decks

Broaden your horizons thru attempting considered one of a type tarot decks. Each deck has a totally specific power and might attraction to wonderful components of your individual. Get notion from particular decks to locate the deck that extraordinary suits your religious journey.

Add a personal contact to your deck.

Make your tarot deck a private expression of your adventure. Add notes, draw symbols or stitch particular pockets. Personalizing your deck creates a deeper connection and specific which means.

Treat your deck with care.

Handle your tarot deck with care. Do now not allow others to use it carelessly and most effective lend it to human beings you recall. Your deck is a sacred tool that consists of your electricity, so treat it with top notch care.

Developing a Tarot Meditation with the Deck

The connection you've got were given built collectively with your tarot deck is the essential factor to deeper insights and transformative memories. Be ready for the subsequent leg of your journey.

Chapter 2: The Number One Symbols Of The Tarot Playing Cards

In the world of Tarot meditation, the symbols at the playing playing cards are the vital component to deeper insights and intuitive information. These symbols are not mere illustrations but have deeper symbolism that wants to be understood.

The Major Arcana is the primary location we will find out. These 22 gambling cards constitute archetypal forces and levels of existence. Each card has a very specific message and symbolizes an element of our individual and collective lifestyles direction.

The Fool's card is the primary of the Major Arcana. Here the idiot symbolizes the start of a journey, childlike take into account and the infinite opportunities that lie ahead. He encourages human beings to discover lifestyles without prejudice or worry.

The magician symbolizes creativity and the capability to show goals into truth. The raised hand connects heaven and earth and reminds us that we are the architects of our very own future.

The High Priestess embodies intuition and statistics. Wrapped in a veil, it symbolizes the depths of mystery and the subconscious. She encourages us to pay attention to our internal voice and embody the strength of intuition.

Ruler represents femininity and fertility. She symbolizes the maternal detail that gives safety and safety. Rulers (rulers) remind us that we have to deal with ourselves and deal with ourselves with love and care.

The ruler symbolizes authority and form. With his stick in his hand, he symbolizes the capacity to take responsibility and create a solid foundation. The ruler reminds us that a clean shape paves the manner to achievement.

The fanatics signify picks and relationships: they stand amongst people and their father or mother angel, reminding them to make alternatives out of love and to fee their relationships with others.

The chariot represents assertiveness and control. The chariot guides the horse in a particular direction, reminding us that desires can be completed thru clean motive and situation.

Justice symbolizes stability and fairness. With a scale in her fingers, she reminds us that our moves have effects and that justice is a important trouble of existence.

The hermit symbolizes introspection and contemplated picture. With lantern in hand, she encourages us to looking for the inner slight and strive for deeper understanding. The Hermit teaches that records is acquired through self-pondered image.

The wheel of fortune symbolizes the circle of life. It reminds us that the whole thing in lifestyles modifications and that we have the energy to steer the course of our lives.

Power represents inner power and compassion. The female and the lion represent the strength of affection and the potential to overcome troubles with staying strength and statistics.

The prisoner embodies catch 22 situation and internal blockage. He reminds us that maximum of the constraints we are going through are self-created and that liberation often begins from indoors.

The tower symbolizes alternate and upheaval. A destroyed tower represents the disintegrate of an old shape, making room for a few element new. Towers remind us that alternate is often inevitable and leads us to growth.

Stars represent wish and notion. They remind us that there's light even in darkish times and that we ought to recognition on our dreams and goals.

The moon represents intuition and the subconscious. The degrees of the moon characterize the special levels of emotions and the want to delve deeper into one's private emotions.

The sun symbolizes strength and pride of life. The glowing slight reminds us to live life to the fullest and focus at the super.

Judgment represents judgment and rebirth. The resurrection of a person symbolizes a brand new starting and the opportunity to check from past mistakes.

The world represents perfection and fulfillment. The dancing discern within the center symbolizes the combination of all factors of lifestyles and the very last touch of a full-size journey.

In addition to the Major Arcana, there are the Minor Arcana, which might be divided into four colored tarot suites: the Cups, Wands, Swords and Pentacles.

The cups represent feelings and relationships. The Cups constitute feelings and relationships and mirror our personal emotions and our relationships with others.

The group of workers represents power and motion. It represents our stress and the manner we pursue our dreams.

The sword symbolizes questioning and communique. It represents how we specific our mind and the way easy our highbrow methods are.

The coins constitute materials and budget. They constitute our connection to the physical international and the way we manipulate our sources.

In the world of tarot gambling cards, know-how the number one symbols is crucial. Each card tells a completely unique story and offers the critical factor to self-reflection and spiritual enlightenment. Take time to find out the symbols, look at their meanings, and use them as courses for your tarot meditation adventure.

The Meaning of the Major Arcana

The Major Arcana of the Tarot is a group of twenty-two gambling gambling playing cards that constitute archetypal forces and additives of lifestyles. These playing playing cards provide deep insights into non secular improvement and numerous components of life beyond regular enjoy.

The Fool's card workplace work the begin of the Major Arcana. The Fool represents unyielding do not forget inside the unknown and the braveness to embark on a journey without know-how the nice route. This card encourages us to find out lifestyles with an open thoughts.

The magician represents the creative energy inner us. It shows that we've were given the power to reveal our desires into truth. The Magician reminds us that we've got the gear and assets to form our destiny.

The High Priestess embodies instinct and information. Wrapped in a veil, it symbolizes the thriller and depths of the unconscious. The card encourages us to be aware about our inner voice and depend upon our unconscious information.

The ruler represents femininity and fertility. As a mother determine, she reminds us to attend to ourselves and deal with ourselves with love. This card invites us to discover nourishing factors within ourselves.

The ruler symbolizes authority and form. With the scepter in his hand, he symbolizes the capability to take obligation and create a solid basis. The ruler reminds us that a clear shape paves the manner to fulfillment.

The fanatics represent picks and relationships; They stand among humans and their father or mother angel and remind us to make picks out of affection and to price our relationships with others.

The chariot represents assertiveness and control. The chariot steers the horse in a positive route and reminds us that a clean will and vicinity will lead us on the direction to success.

Justice symbolizes balance and equity. With a scale in her arms, she reminds us that our actions have effects and that justice is a relevant detail of lifestyles.

The hermit symbolizes introspection and contemplated photo. With a lantern in hand, she urges us to are searching for the internal light and attempt for deeper understanding. The Hermit teaches that statistics is received through self-mirrored picture.

The wheel of fortune symbolizes the circle of existence. It reminds us that the whole thing in lifestyles modifications and that we've the strength to steer the route of our lives.

Power represents internal electricity and compassion. The girl and the lion represent the electricity of love and the potential to conquer problems with staying energy and understanding.

The prisoner embodies downside and internal blockage. He reminds us that the diverse obstacles we are going via are self-created and that liberation frequently starts offevolved offevolved from inner.

The tower symbolizes alternate and upheaval. A destroyed tower represents the collapse of an vintage structure, making room for a few factor new. Towers remind us that exchange is frequently inevitable and leads us to growth.

The stars constitute need and concept. They remind us that there is moderate even in darkish instances and that we need to attention on our desires and desires.

The moon represents instinct and the unconscious. The stages of the moon represent the wonderful degrees of emotions and the want to delve deeper into one's very non-public feelings.

The sun symbolizes electricity and pride of life. The shining moderate reminds us to stay lifestyles to the fullest and attention at the amazing.

The judgment symbolizes judgment and rebirth. The resurrection of someone symbolizes a present day beginning and the opportunity to study from beyond mistakes. The worldwide represents perfection and success. The dancing decide inside the middle symbolizes the combination of all factors of existence and the finishing touch of a massive adventure.

Each Major Arcana card tells a very specific story and gives us deep insights into precise factors of our lives. They are not most effective a divination tool, but as an alternative a gateway to our very non-public data and development of our non secular route. Use the Major Arcana as a key to self-reflected photograph and a manual in your Tarot meditation journey.

Chapter 3: The Meaning of the Minor Arcana

Another fascinating financial ruin opens in the worldwide of Tarot: the Minor Arcana. It includes four suits or tarot suites: the Cup, the Wand, the Sword and the Coin. Each of those suites represents a first rate vicinity of life or an trouble of our being.

The cups symbolize feelings and relationships. They replicate our internal maximum emotions and the way we connect to others. From satisfaction and like to unhappiness and loss, the cups replicate a big style of human emotions.

The frame of people symbolizes power and movement. It represents our energy and the manner we pursue our desires. The staff symbolizes creativity and assertiveness and encourages us to reap this and positioned mind into motion.

The sword symbolizes questioning and communication. It shows how we specific our thoughts and how clean our intellectual techniques are. The sword represents every truth and venture, encouraging us to harness the energy of our spirit.

Coins represent substances and charge range. They reflect our connection to the bodily world and the way we control our belongings. Coins remind us of the significance of stability and reason in our lives.

In the Cup combination, the Ace of Cups represents the mystical Cup, the supply of all feelings. The essence of affection, compassion and emotional wealth is contained on this card.

The 2 of Cups represents partnership and harmony; the 2 cups are united and represent the capability for mutual enchantment and deep connection.

The Three of Cups represents pleasure and community; the three have amusing collectively and emphasize the importance of shared reviews and absolutely glad togetherness.

The Four of Cups symbolizes self-pondered photo and internal exploration. The determine with its again grew to end up indicates that there are instances on the equal time as one must pause to understand one's very personal inner wishes.

The Five of Cups represents loss and grief. The fallen cups represent disillusioned expectations, at the same time as the 2 upright cups represent wish and the opportunity of a today's beginning.

The Six of Cups symbolizes nostalgia and reminiscences. The characters look returned on beyond research and discover ways to draw energy from the beyond.

The Seven of Cups symbolizes desires and imagination. It encourages the individual to pursue vision and use the innovative power of imagination.

The eight of Cups represents the preference for change and the pursuit of religious growth. She leaves the 8 upright cups to discover deeper meanings.

The Nine of Cups represents success and happiness; Nine cups suggest the fulfillment of private goals and desires.

The Ten of Cups symbolizes emotional happiness and contentment; the idyllic scene with ten upright goblets emphasizes abundance and success on an emotional diploma.

The Ace of Wands symbolizes a extremely-current starting entire of energy and exuberance. The upright body of people represents modern pursuits and the capability for a robust begin.

The Two of Wands represents planning and desire making. Looking to the horizon symbolizes the exploration of new possibilities and the recognition of possibilities.

Wand 3 symbolizes increase and boom. The determine seems into the gap and alerts that making an investment in lengthy-term desires will bear fruit.

Wand 4 represents balance and success. Wand four paperwork a celebratory form that shows the success of goals and superb consequences.

Wand 5 symbolizes battle and mission. The characters fight for manage, indicating the want for cooperation and compromise. The Six of Wands symbolizes reputation and fulfillment. A powerful appearance on horseback suggests public reputation and admiration.

The 7 of Wands represents resistance and assertiveness. The man or woman defends his feature and reminds us that there are instances whilst fortitude is vital.

The eight of Wands symbolizes rapid exchange and dynamism; The eight sticks fly brief via the air and represent development and prolonged development.

The 9 of Wands symbolizes resilience and staying power. It represents internal electricity that stays however issues.

Rod 10 represents overload and burden. It indicates that this character is wearing a heavy burden and that it is time to delegate duty and lighten the load.

The Ace of Swords indicates a smooth spiritual step forward. The upright sword pierces the clouds and symbolizes the electricity of clear thinking and assertiveness.

The Two of Swords symbolizes desire making and internal warfare. The character holds swords in his hand and weighs precise alternatives.

The 1/3 sword symbolizes heartbreak and loss. The swords pierce the coronary heart and constitute emotional pain and sadness.

The Four of Swords symbolizes peace and calmness. The decide resting underneath the cover reminds us that rest is essential for regeneration.

The Five of Swords represents war and defeat. It indicates that the man or woman has conflicts and that no longer all conflicts may be acquired.

The Six of Swords symbolizes transition and change. The character is crossing calm waters, indicating a transition to calm waters.

The Seven of Swords symbolizes deception and foxy. The decide sneaks away, reminding us that not the whole thing is as it appears.

The eighth sword represents imprisonment and limited imaginative and prescient. The individual is surrounded with the resource of eight swords, which represent self-imposed limitations.

The Nine of Swords symbolizes fear and worry. The man or woman is surrounded via nine swords, indicating that worry frequently arises in a single's very personal thoughts.

The Ten of Swords symbolizes the prevent of painful topics. The decide is placed underneath the Ten of Swords, indicating the prevent of a disturbing cycle.

The Ace of Five represents cloth success and abundance. The upright coin symbolizes the begin of monetary praise and safety.

The Two of Pentacles represents balance and flexibility. The decide juggles cash, indicating the need for skillful use of belongings.

The Three of Pentacles represents teamwork and cooperation; 3 human beings work collectively on a challenge and therefore show appreciation for joint efforts.

The Four of Pentacles represents preserving immediately to possessions. The characters preserve four coins that remind them of the significance of being open to change.

The Five of Pentacles symbolizes scarcity and uncertainty. The man or woman is inside the snow, indicating that assistance is frequently to be had if one seeks it.

The Six of Pentacles symbolizes giving and receiving. The person offers generously and indicates a balance of power and resources.

The Seven of Pentacles represents patience and funding. The figure waits for the fruit to ripen, indicating that right topics take time.

The 8 of Pentacles symbolizes know-how and strength of will. The man or woman is absorbed in his artwork, reminding us that dedication ends in mastery.

The 9 of the pentagram symbolizes independence and self-sufficiency. The discern gambling the harvest by myself represents personal success and freedom. The ten on the coin represents cloth wealth and circle of relatives inheritance. The parent reputation within the the front of a residence reminds us that achievement is frequently generational.

The Minor Arcana provides an in depth map of the human experience. It shows the form of existence, from relationships and behavior to thoughts and fabric subjects. Use the Minor Arcana as a manual to understand and consciously form the correct components of your lifestyles.

The Meaning of the Four Tarot Suites

The international of tarot playing cards starts offevolved offevolved with 4 tremendous tarot suites: the Chalice, the Wand, the Sword and the Coin. Each of these pairs represents a completely specific difficulty of human existence and offers us deep insights into superb elements of our enjoy.

Cups - feelings and interpersonal relationships:

The cup is a photo of deep emotions and interpersonal relationships. It displays our personal emotional existence and indicates our connection to others. From pleasure and prefer to sadness and loss, the cup lets in us to check out the depths of our feelings.

Wands - Energy and Action

The group of workers represents power, passion and movement. He is the the use of stress within the returned of our actions and initiatives. When the employees appears in an interpretation, it indicates the power to set topics in movement and take progressive initiative.

Sword - Thinking and Communication:

The sword represents easy wondering and communication. It suggests the sharpness of mind and the way you precise your self. In warfare conditions, the sword can recommend the want to provide readability and sell open conversation.

Coins - cloth and financial:

Coins constitute the bodily worldwide, fabric wealth and financial topics. They replicate how we manipulate our sources, are looking for material protection, and find out our place inside the global.

Ass.

The Ace in every tarot represents new beginnings and the ability for increase. The Ace of Cups symbolizes a new beginning in emotional relationships. The Ace of Wands brings new strength and a wave of creative possibilities. The Ace of Swords symbolizes a religious soar in advance. The Ace of Five represents the begin of cloth prosperity.

2 to ten.

The gambling gambling playing cards from 2 to ten in every pair represent first-rate levels of development and disturbing situations. Each variety brings a completely unique dynamic and depth to the cardboard's that means.

Court playing cards.

The court docket gambling playing cards Page, Knight, Queen and King represent nice personalities and energies. The Page represents hobby and studying, the Knight represents passion and interest, the Queen represents emotional intelligence, and the King represents authority and balance.

Interpretation.

When interpreting the Tarot Suite, it is essential to look the playing gambling playing cards within the context of the question or topic. The combination of gambling playing cards can offer subtle nuances and deeper perception right into a state of affairs. The feature of the gambling playing cards inside the laying system additionally may be taken into consideration to provide greater statistics about timing and urgency.

Practical recommendations

Connect with the electricity: Before a tarot studying, discover a quiet vicinity and take time to center yourself. Connect with the energy of the gambling playing cards and open your mind to the message they are in search of to hold to you.

Ask Clear Questions: Ask easy and concise questions to manual the gambling cards. The extra unique your question is, the clearer the gambling cards' solution could be.

Pay attention to ordinary patterns: If a particular card or pattern seems in unique interpretations, be aware it. Repetitive styles can suggest important topics or inclinations for your existence.

Trust your intuition: The cards provide shape, but your instinct additionally plays an essential function. Trust how the gambling cards have an impact on you and what feelings and mind they evoke.

Keep a religious magazine: Record your tarot readings and the insights you advantage from them in a mag. This lets in you to music your progress, select out ordinary troubles and assist your intuition.

The Tarot playing cards are a fascinating key to better understanding our emotional depth, our progressive energy, our clarity of thoughts and our fabric worldwide. Using this manual as a compass, you can flip the Tarot gambling cards into your private guide and advantage a comprehensive perspective on your lifestyles.

Chapter 4: Preparation and Attunement to Meditation

Meditation is a effective exercise that let you locate calm, clarity and internal concord. To revel in the total intensity and impact of Tarot meditation, aware training and attunement is essential. In this bankruptcy you'll discover ways to optimally prepare to your meditation and create a harmonious environment in your non secular adventure.

1. Find a Quiet Place:

Find a quiet location where you may not be disturbed. A location that radiates peace and calm allows the attention and deepening of your meditation.

2. Set up your area:

Design your meditation area consciously. You can use candles, incense, or important oils to create a pleasing environment. Choose symbols that have a totally unique which means that that for you and which you would really like to fee with religious energy.

three. Comfortable garb:

Wear free, cushty garb that does not restrict your movements. This promotes a snug posture and lets in you to engage in meditation more without issues.

four. Physical education:

Sit or lie down in a snug position. Make high quality your backbone is right now to permit for optimum energy drift. Before meditating, loosen up your shoulders and neck to release anxiety.

5. Breathing techniques:

Start via using taking a few aware breaths to relax. Deep breaths calm the worried tool and put together you to transport deeper into your meditation. Breathe inner and out slowly and gently, focusing your hobby on the breath.

6. Attunement with Tarot Cards:

Look on the tarot playing cards you chose for your meditation. Let your gaze slide gently over the symbols and take in the power of the gambling playing cards. Imagine your self entering into a talk with these symbols.

7. Set a smooth purpose:

Set a clear reason for your meditation. What do you want to study or understand? Your intention gives your meditation clean course and allows you to specially address subjects or questions.

8th. Visualization:

Use the strength of visualization to get within the mood for meditation. Imagine a defensive energy surrounding you. Visualize your self entering into a sacred area illuminated through the symbols of the tarot gambling cards.

nine. Sound and tune:

Use calming sounds or meditation tune to manual the environment. Soft music or nature sounds can calm your senses and energize the meditation room.

10. Timing:

Set a low-fee time to your meditation. It isn't always essential to meditate for a long term; however it's far essential to exercise regularly. Maybe start with 10 to fifteen minutes and increase the length as desired.

Eleven. Mindful Quitting:

End the meditation mindfully. Take a deep breath and sense yourself consciously returning to the room. Close the meditation by way of the usage of announcing thanks and taking tremendous strength into your regular life.

Through aware steerage and attunement, you can deepen your meditation and enjoy the energies of the tarot gambling cards in a profound way. Let this manner manual you and permit the symbols to serve you on your religious journey.

Breathing for Deep Meditation

The paintings of meditation lie no longer handiest in quiet contemplation, but additionally in aware regulation and awareness at the breath. Breathing is a effective bridge amongst body and mind. This financial ruin introduces numerous breathing strategies to deepen meditation and create a deeper reference to the internal self.

Conscious respiratory

Begin your meditation by using manner of turning into privy to your breath. Notice how the breath flows into the nostril, fills the frame after which evenly flows out once more. Find a natural rhythm in your breathing and consciously be aware the manner it invigorates you.

Deep abdominal respiration:

Sit or lie down in a comfortable characteristic. Place one hand to your stomach and the alternative to your chest. Breathe deeply into your belly, and whilst you experience it developing, breathe out slowly. This approach promotes deeper relaxation and calm, even respiratory.

Counting technique:

Count in time along aspect your breath to deepen attention. Inhale and be counted to 4; maintain your breath four instances; exhale four instances. Repeat this cycle numerous instances. This technique now not handiest promotes mindfulness, but moreover calms the go together with the drift of breath.

Hold breath:

After taking a deep breath, maintain your breath for a while and then exhale slowly. Holding your breath promotes internal calm and allows you interest at the triumphing 2d. Start with quick poses and grade by grade extend them.

5. Die Wechselatmung (Nadi Shodhana):

Alternately close to the left and right nostrils collectively along with your hands and breathe outside and inside through the open nostril. Balances the mind hemispheres and promotes concord eventually of the electricity system.

6. Ujjayi-Atmung:

Inhale thru your nostril, inhale gently through your larynx and make a slight sound. This technique, moreover known as "sea sound," promotes relaxation and interest.

Breathing declaration:

Don't manage your respiratory, without a doubt have a have a look at your breathing. Let the breath flow certainly and attention at the way it feels. When a concept entails mind, gently deliver your hobby once more to the breath. This method promotes mindfulness and inner silence.

Atem-Mantra:

Connect the breath with a chilled mantra. As you breathe in, repeat high-quality phrases or brief phrases in your head. As you breathe out, allow flow into of horrible thoughts. This method lets in calm the thoughts and increase excellent energy.

Respiration cycles:

Imagine your breath circulating and flowing through your body. Breathe deeply into your stomach, supply your breath into your chest and over again into your stomach as you breathes out. Visualizing this cycle creates a deeper connection.

Breathing and Tarot Symbols:

Connect respiratory with the symbols of the tarot gambling cards. Imagine that with each breath you are taking within the energy of the selected card. Allow the symbols to go with the flow via your frame as you breathe and enjoy their transformative electricity.

These breathing carrying sports activities offer special strategies to deepening meditation. Try specific techniques and notice which suits extraordinary for you. By consciously combining respiratory and meditation, you could delve deeper into your inner self and revel in the non secular know-how of the tarot playing playing cards.

Chapter 5: Visualization Techniques in the Tarot Meditation Process

The energy of imagination is a effective tool at the route of meditation. Visualization can redecorate the symbols of tarot playing playing playing cards into colorful pics that penetrate deep into the unconscious. This financial smash explores visualization strategies that growth the system of Tarot meditation and create a deeper connection with the gambling playing cards.

Symbolic journey:

Imagine diving into the arena of tarot playing playing cards. Imagine taking walks down a direction protected with map symbols. Walk consciously through those symbols and watch them come to life. This method permits you to expand a private dating with the gambling playing cards.

Tarot Garden:

Create a lawn in your creativeness with every card within the tarot represented. Explore this garden, touch the flora of the Chalice, sense the power of the Staff, revel in the statistics of the Sword, and taste the cloth wealth of the Coin. This visible garden can be a deliver of idea and reflection.

The 1/3 Tarot mandala:

Imagine that the tarot playing playing cards turn out to be the picture of a mandala. Observe the symmetry and special colorings due to the fact the mandala takes shape to your mind's eye. Harmonious placement of playing playing cards promotes readability and stability.

Card interaction:

Visualize how the tarot gambling playing cards engage with each top notch. The gambling playing cards can circulate, communicate with each distinctive and form new pictures. Gain a deeper knowledge of the connections among the gambling cards and find out their reminiscences.

Cards as mirrors:

Think of the tarot gambling gambling cards as mirrors that reflect your inner self. Imagine searching into each card and the way the symbols inside it have an effect on you. This lets in for deep self-knowledge and religious reflected photograph.

Maps and dream trips:

Use the tarot playing playing cards as the important thing on your dream adventure. Visualize yourself immersed in a selected card scene and experiencing the electricity inside it. This opens up new dimensions of belief and famous hidden insights.

Guided card meditation:

Let your inner guide guide you through the symbolism of the tarot playing cards. Imagine that you are being guided by manner of using a clever character inside the various situations that the gambling playing cards represent. This guided meditation will offer you with deep insights.

Card Transformation:

Imagine the tarot playing cards converting in your mind. The card can alternate colour, shape, or address a super photo. This symbolizes exchange and increase to your non secular route.

nine. Area the tarot symbols into your frame:

Imagine that the symbols of the tarot playing cards seem in your frame. The cup represents the emotions to your heart, the group of workers represents the energy on your arms, the sword represents the clean mind to your head and the coin represents the prosperity in your belly. This visualization permits the deep integration of the Tarot strength internal you.

Think of the playing gambling playing cards as rays of mild:

Visualize the tarot playing cards as great rays of moderate coming down toward you. Feel how each mild fills you with its particular power. This serves as a cleansing and invigorating technique.

These visualization techniques open up a global of creative possibilities for bringing the tarot cards to existence in meditation. Experiment with one of a kind techniques, use your imagination and open the door to deeper facts. Through the power of visualization, the symbols of the tarot gambling gambling cards can become a residing companion on your religious adventure.

The Art of Conscious Relaxation

In a worldwide this is regularly worrying and demanding, the artwork of aware rest becomes an essential skills. This financial disaster is dedicated to developing conscious relaxation strategies that promote deeper stability, internal peace, and intellectual clarity.

Basics of aware relaxation

Conscious relaxation starts with the preference to provide yourself a destroy. It is an act of self-care that balances frame, mind and soul. The first step is to permit yourself to loosen up without feeling accountable.

Mindful respiration:

Breathing is the important thing to rest. Mindful respiratory can help lessen stress and create a aware connection with your breath. Sit clearly, near your eyes and cognizance on the herbal float of your respiratory. Breathe inner and out deeply and revel in your muscle corporations relax.

Progressive Muscle Relaxation:

This approach includes tensing a specific muscle employer and then consciously exciting it. Start at your toes and slowly loosen up up on your head. It relieves tension throughout the body and promotes deep relaxation.

Visualization strategies:

Use your imagination to create an area of peace and concord. Close your eyes and imagine a place that represents peace and rest to you. Imagine every component of this location and create an oasis on your thoughts.

Meditation for relaxation:

Meditation is an powerful manner to lighten up. Sit in a snug function and consciousness for your breathing or use a guided meditation to calm your mind and collect a rustic of internal peace.

Yoga and stretching:

Physical sports like yoga and mild stretching can help relieve physical tension and calm the thoughts. Practice yoga poses and stretches regularly to increase your flexibility and decrease pressure.

Importance of breaks in day by day life:

Make a aware try to include breaks into your ordinary lifestyles. Stand up, stretch, and breathe deeply as you determine. These short breaks can help reduce stress stages and improve concentration.

Aromatherapy:

Use crucial oils to create a non violent atmosphere. Lavender, chamomile, and bergamot are examples of scents that sell rest. Add them to aroma lamps or baths, or use them in a material and inhale at the same time as exciting.

Digital detox:

Reduce the time you spend on virtual devices. Constant get proper of entry to to statistics and sensory overload from video display units may be disturbing. Take ordinary time an extended way from digital gadgets to sell intellectual calm.

The role of nature:

Relax in nature. A stroll in a park, with the useful resource of the sea or in a wooded area can be glowing and calming. Natural environments help divert recognition from demanding mind.

Self-mirrored photo and relaxation:

Reflect on your self and regularly have a look at your priorities. Identify stress-inflicting factors and boom strategies to cope with them. This promotes conscious residing and strengthens the capacity to consciously relax.

Conscious rest strategies are a lifelong technique that includes mindfulness, self-love and the conscious care of one's non-public properly-being. By incorporating those strategies into each day existence, you could benefit a kingdom of internal calm that now not only reduces pressure however additionally promotes a deeper reference to one's self.

Meditation with Tarot Cards - a step-by way of-step manual

The fusion of meditation and tarot playing playing cards creates a effective platform for non-public increase, mirrored image and religious reputation. In this chapter, we are able to find out an in depth step-with the useful resource of-step guide to meditating with tarot playing playing cards to attach greater deeply with the intuitive statistics of tarot cards.

Choose a tarot card:

Start thru choosing the tarot card you need to meditate on. You can choose a card that resonates with you or create a deck that addresses a specific query or hassle consider.

Find a quiet region to meditate:

Find a quiet location wherein you could loosen up without being disturbed. Light candles, use essential oils, or play smooth song to create a cushty environment.

Sit or lie down with out trouble:

Find a relaxing role. You can each sit or lie down. Keep your decrease again proper away just so the power can go with the flow optimally.

4 respiratory sporting sports activities to alter your thoughts:

Start through consciously taking a few breaths to get yourself within the proper mood. Breathe deeply inner and out out of your stomach. Let your breath go together with the go along with the flow calmly and flippantly and calm your mind.

Look on the tarot card you chose:

Focus your interest on the tarot card in the front of you. Let your gaze slide gently over the symbols, colors and data. Consciously experience the energy of the card.

Clear purpose:

Set a clean purpose for meditation. What do you want to analyze from the Tarot playing cards? What questions do you want to reply? A smooth reason directs your interest and opens the distance for deeper insights.

Visualize the symbols:

Close your eyes and don't forget the tarot card symbols coming to life. Immerse yourself in the scene of the card and bear in mind yourself interacting with the power it includes.

Focus on the person statistics:

Deepen your meditation by means of way of using focusing on the person facts of the gambling gambling cards. Look at every image, every form and each color. Pay interest to the emotions and thoughts that stand up.

Ask the card a question:

Ask the tarot playing playing cards questions on your current life situation, choices, inner worrying conditions, and plenty of others. Allow the answers to drift intuitively for your popularity.

10. Stay in silence:

Let the meditation result in silence. Just be there and allow your self to experience the strength of the tarot playing gambling playing cards. Be open to the impulses that arise from internal you.

Record your revel in:

After meditating, file your revel in. Write down which symbols were specially gift, which feelings arose and which insights you received. A meditation magazine can be useful.

Complete 12 breathing wearing events:

At the stop of the meditation, take some aware breaths. Breathe deeply to combine the insights gained and breathe out to allow move. Feel yourself growing from meditation with sparkling power and clarity.

Meditation with tarot playing cards is a effective exercise that brings the deep information of the gambling cards into your attention. With this step-with the resource of-step guide, you may be part of deeply with the symbols and energies of the Tarot cards and beautify your non secular journey.

Chapter 6: The Importance of Colors and Symbols in Meditation

The worldwide of meditation is rich in symbols and colors which can provide deep insights into the internal self. This economic destroy explores the importance of colors and logos in meditation and how their conscious integration can enhance the spiritual journey.

Color psychology in meditation

Colors have a sturdy have an impact on on our feelings and our thoughts. In meditation, positive hues can evoke certain moods. For instance, white represents purity and clarity, on the equal time as blue is regularly related to calm and accept as true with. Recognize the psychology of colours and consciously choose shades steady together with your meditation purpose.

Red power:

Red is the shade of ardour and electricity. Use purple in meditation to draw to your inner electricity. Imagine that a purple moderate envelops you and flows strength into you, strengthening your power and life strain.

Orange - creativity:

Orange represents creativity and emotional expression. Use orange in meditation to activate your modern energy. Imagine a warmness orange pass flowing thru your modern middle and horrifying you.

Yellow brightness:

Yellow is the shade of brightness and spirit. In meditation, yellow clears the thoughts and promotes highbrow clarity. Imagine the wonderful yellow dispelling the darkness and bringing slight into your focus.

Green heals:

Green is related to recovery and harmony. In meditation, inexperienced moderate can be used to heal emotional wounds and create a experience of balance. Imagine a inexperienced mist surrounding you, bringing restoration to every part of your being.

Blue Serenity:

Blue symbolizes serenity and peace. In meditation, blue can be used to calm the thoughts and create an atmosphere of stillness. Imagine how the mild blue surrounds you and fills each breath with internal peace.

Violet Spirituality:

Purple represents spirituality and intuition. Use the shade pink in meditation to reinforce your spiritual talents. Imagine a violet air of mystery connecting you to better tiers of recognition and unlocking intuitive understanding.

White purification:

White represents purity and readability. Use white in meditation to loose your self from all burdens. Imagine white mild flowing thru your being, cleaning all negativity and making area for latest electricity.

Symbols in meditation:

Symbols have non secular which means in lots of cultures. During meditation, symbols function a focal point for deep insights. Use symbols which have personal which means that that, in conjunction with: E.G. The Ohm signal or the Yin-Yang photograph.

Elements of Nature:

Incorporate natural elements which includes plant life, wooden, and water into your meditation. These symbols have a herbal strength and promote a deeper reference to the earth and its herbal cycles.

Symbols which might be particular to you:

Create symbols which have personal meaning for you. This can be a shape, a sample or perhaps your very personal handwriting. These non-public symbols create a effective connection for your inner self.

Mandala-Meditation:

Use a mandala as a seen focal detail for meditation. The mandala may be a sacred geometric determine or a pattern which you have drawn your self. Look on the facts of the mandala and calm your mind.

Spiritual symbols:

Incorporate extraordinary non secular symbols into your workout. This can be a spiritual photo, an archetype or a sacred expression. Use them as a gateway to deeper religious reviews. The conscious use of colours and logos in meditation opens up a global of symbolic communication and religious facts. Incorporating those factors into your meditation workout no longer most effective lets in you to gain deeper internal yourself, however moreover lets in you to revel in a wealthy and big religious adventure.

Explore Your Intuition

Intuition is a effective pressure that allows us look deeper inner ourselves and tap right into a information that transcends cause. This chapter addresses exploring one's very very very own intuition as an essential detail of self-development. It gives sensible guidance for data and strengthening your internal voice.

Develop recollect on your private intuition

Trusting your very personal intuition is the key to successful exploration. Recognize that intuition isn't always primarily based totally on rational evidence, but alternatively on deep inner belief. Start with the resource of trusting your instinct and accepting it as a deliver of steering.

Mindfulness and introspection:

Mindfulness is the first step to exploring your instinct. Make time for normal contemplated image. Observe your mind, feelings and reactions to 1-of-a-kind conditions. This mindfulness will assist you recognize the subtle indicators of instinct.

Find the silence:

Intuition regularly speaks in silence. To reduce the noise of regular existence, regularly are looking for moments of peace and quiet. In the silence you'll be aware of the quiet suggestions of your internal voice.

Explore your intuition:

Intuition is a effective tool of instinct. Pay interest to the sensations to your stomach. Intuition can take vicinity itself as moderate soreness or top notch warmth. Learn to interpret the ones subtle frame sensations.

Keep a dream diary:

Dreams are frequently a window to intuition. Keep a dream mag to document and examine your goals. Dreams often consist of symbolic messages and will permit you to gain deeper notion into your feelings and disturbing situations.

Creative expression:

Creativity is a bridge to intuition. Use your creativity through drawing, writing, dancing or making track. Creative expression opens doors to deeper tiers of cognizance and allows instinct to emerge in a playful manner.

Thought preventing techniques:

In stressful conditions, it is able to be difficult to apply intuition. Use the idea stopping approach to break the glide of thoughts for a quick time body. Close your eyes, breathe internal and out deeply, then sit down down in stillness and concentrate on your intuition.

Consult your internal know-how:

Consciously ask questions of your internal awareness. Sit in a comfortable us of a and ask smooth, open-ended questions. Then allow your self to concentrate to the answers that come decrease again within the form of pics, emotions and internal voices.

Recognize symbols and characters:

Intuition regularly speaks to you in symbols and symptoms and signs and symptoms. Pay interest to habitual symbols and unusual signs and symptoms and symptoms for your every day life. These can offer you with information approximately vital alternatives and developments.

Use intuitive gear:

Tarot cards, pendulums, and one of a kind intuitive device can be used to boom your instinct. Allow the symbols and energies of those device to show insights to you. They act like mirrors that reflect your internal information.

Trust the method:

Exploring your instinct is an ongoing way. Trust that your instinct will deepen and turn out to be clearer over the years. Also be for the reason that it is regular that you will no longer acquire all of the solutions proper away.

Exploring intuition is a adventure of self-discovery. By being affected character, aware, and open, you can help your internal voice and advantage deeper insights. Intuition is a precious manual for existence.

Chapter 7: The Role of Dreams in Tarot Meditation

Dreams are a gateway to the depths of the unconscious and offer deep insights into the inner self. This monetary destroy explores the charming connection amongst dreams and tarot meditation. Not high-quality will you look at the that means of dreams on this context, but you can additionally accumulate practical commands on the way to contain dream symbols into your tarot card meditations.

The language of goals

Dreams regularly communicate a symbolic language this is hard to decipher. However, information the signs and logos that seem in desires allows us to get proper of entry to deeper layers of the unconscious. Tarot meditation gives a framework for interpreting this symbolic language.

Dream symbols and tarot playing cards

The archetypes and logos of the tarot playing gambling cards frequently find correspondences in our desires. Pay interest to the tarot gambling cards and logos that appear in your dreams. They shape a deeper bridge most of the waking usa and the dream state.

Dream art work as guidance

Before you begin your tarot meditation, take time to consider your dream. Keep a dream magazine to file habitual problems, symbols, and emotions. This preparatory art work creates a conscious connection among your dream experience and the tarot playing gambling cards.

Dream incubation for particular questions

Use the dream incubation technique to get solutions to specific questions. Before you fall asleep, ask your self a question and bear in thoughts receiving the solution to your dream. This machine can open deeper stages of know-how in Tarot meditation.

Incorporate dream symbols into meditation

During Tarot meditation, consciously consider the dream symbols that appeared all through sleep. Imagine how those symbols inside the tarot playing cards come to existence and play an lively function in meditation. This lets in the relationship a number of the dream and the waking united states.

Interpretation of goals with tarot playing cards

Use tarot cards as a device for dream interpretation. Lay out the playing cards and examine them for your dream. Pay hobby to the resonance most of the gambling cards and the dream symbols. The playing cards characteristic a key to discover deeper meanings in dreams.

The feature of feelings

Emotions play an important characteristic in each dreams and tarot meditation. Pay interest to the emotions that arise in the dream and discover how they relate to the tarot cards. Emotional resonance deepens the know-how and which means of the message.

Take a dream walk thru the tarot panorama:

During meditation, accept as true with that you are getting into a dreamscape inspired via the tarot playing playing playing cards. Walk through the ones dreamscapes and produce the tarot symbols to existence. This dream stroll promotes the mixture of dream and tarot meditation.

Lucid dreaming for deeper insights:

Train lucid dreaming techniques to paintings consciously on your desires. This allows you to actively have interaction with tarot cards and dream symbols. Lucid dreaming offers a completely unique possibility to delve deeper into the arena of tarot meditation.

Reflect frequently:

Take the time to often mirror to your Tarot meditations and dream testimonies. Pay interest to how the dream symbolism is pondered in the tarot playing cards and the manner it expands your information. Regular mirrored photo promotes the similarly development of this charming interplay.

The connection amongst goals and Tarot meditation opens up a wealth of non secular insights. Consciously exploring dream symbols in mixture with tarot cards not top notch permits you to delve deeper into your subconscious, however also advantage a broader angle in your non secular adventure.

Overcoming Obstacles - Tips for Successful Meditation

The practice of meditation has many blessings for the body and thoughts, however limitations regularly upward thrust up that stand inside the way of a deep and pleasing meditation workout. This financial ruin addresses the most not unusual boundaries which can upward push up for the duration of meditation and presents sensible tips for overcoming them and effectively working toward the meditation addiction.

Restless Mind:

Tip: Focus your interest and sustained interest on the breath. Start with quick meditation instructions and regularly boom the time. Accept that mind come and circulate and allow them to bypass with out preserving on to them.

Physical pain:

Tip: Find a sitting function this is cushty for you. Try awesome sitting positions and help your self with pillows or blankets. Take deep breaths to launch anxiety and pass as wanted during meditation.

I haven't any time:

Tip: Include brief meditation training for your every day ordinary. They don't continually must be lengthy intervals. Even regular meditation sessions of quick period can also need to have powerful outcomes. Prioritize your meditation time to gain the blessings of meditation.

Impatience:

Tip: Develop endurance with the resource of being privy to the prevailing 2nd. Focus to your respiratory and allow skip of the selection for instant success. The fruits of meditation will encompass time.

Sleep fashion:

Tip: Meditation isn't an opportunity to sleep, but if fatigue happens during meditation, constantly try to sit down down in an upright role and set off the mind via conscious respiration. Also keep in thoughts meditating at a one-of-a-kind time of day.

Distractions:

Tip: Create a quiet meditation region and reduce distractions. Use earplugs or an eye fixed consistent masks if vital. Accept distractions with out judgment and lightly deliver your hobby decrease decrease returned to the meditation.

Self-doubt:

Tip: Accept that self-doubt is normal. Acknowledge them, but do not come to be aware about with them. Meditation is an area of boom and self-knowledge, now not perfection.

Unusual sensations:

Tip: When an ugly feeling arises, examine it cautiously without becoming emotionally connected to it. Accept that sensations come and pass. Focus your hobby at the remarkable factors of meditation.

I do not sense inspired to meditate:

Tip: Set easy dreams on your meditation. Be easy approximately why you are meditating and what blessings you expect from meditation. To live advocated, take into account the effective changes meditation can bring for your life.

Lack of normal:

Tip: Set a meditation habitual with a fixed time and place. Routines help combine meditation into normal life and make it part of your lifestyles.

Overcoming boundaries to meditation requires mindfulness, reputation, and non-prevent exercise. By following those hints, you can't pleasant conquer the maximum commonplace demanding situations, but moreover combine a fulfillment and notable meditation into your everyday life.

Chapter 8: Tarot Meditation in Exquisite Areas of Life

Tarot meditation is a effective way to shed mild on diverse elements of existence and gain religious insights. This economic damage gives with the great areas of life wherein Tarot meditation can be achieved. It gives sensible steering and belief into how tarot playing playing playing cards may be used to advantage deeper notion in various areas of life, from relationships to profession and personal improvement.

Relationships 1:

INSTRUCTIONS: Choose tarot playing playing cards that constitute you and your companion. Meditate on the ones cards and bear in mind how your energies flow into each distinctive." Ask questions which includes "What contributes to harmony in our relationship?" and "How are we able to recognize each different better?

Career and assignment:

Here's a way to do it: Draw 3 tarot gambling cards that constitute the past, present and destiny of your professional situation. Consider how the cards relate for your professional career. What stressful conditions have you ever overcome inside the beyond, what possibilities do you study now and how can you put together for the destiny?" Ask.

Finance:

Guide: Focus on tarot playing cards that want to do with rate variety, together with: B. The coin suite. Ask approximately economic demanding conditions and opportunities. Meditate on the cards and ask, "How can I enhance my financial state of affairs? How can I beautify my financial state of affairs?

Health and properly-being:

GUIDE: Use the tarot cards to shed slight in your bodily and intellectual health. Ask approximately the reasons of contamination and the manner you can heal yourself.

Choose a card that represents fitness and fitness to you and meditate on its that means.

Self-assist:

Here's the manner to do it: Draw a card that represents your contemporary degree of lifestyles. Ask about regions of personal growth. Meditate on the card and ask, "What traits do I need to increase to reap my whole functionality?"

Spiritual Growth:

Choose a tarot card that represents a non secular subject matter, at the side of: B. "Hierophant" or "High Priest". Ask approximately your spiritual path and the lessons the universe has in keep for you. Meditate on the cardboard and ask for religious increase.

Family and home:

GUIDE: Use tarot playing cards to understand own family and domestic dynamics. Ask about harmony, battle and opportunities for improvement. Meditate on the playing cards and ask, "How can I construct a harmonious domestic?" Ask.

Creativity and self-expression:

Instructions: Choose a card that represents creativity and self-expression, on the facet of the Chalice Suite. Ask about your innovative power and the manner you could launch it. Meditate on the cardboard and ask, "What modern-day capacity is inner me?" Ask.

9 Social surroundings:

Here's the way it genuinely works: Draw a card that represents your social environment. Ask about your friendships, social connections and networks. Meditate on the card and ask the subsequent questions.

10. Future possibilities:

Here's a manner to do it: Choose a tarot card that symbolizes the electricity of your destiny development. Ask about the possibilities and demanding situations. Meditate on the card and ask, "What awaits me inside the destiny and the manner can I prepare for it?"

Tarot meditation offers a bendy possibility to advantage deeper insights into unique regions of life. By consciously incorporating the tarot gambling playing cards into meditation, one cannot most effective gain a clear view of numerous elements of existence, however furthermore practical advice for non-public improvement.

Integrating meditation into each day existence

Integrating meditation into ordinary lifestyles is vital so you can definitely take benefit of the wonderful results of meditation. This economic disaster gives practical commands and insights into the manner to smoothly combine meditation into regular existence. From morning rituals to taking quick breaks at a few degree in the day, we are going to find out one among a type strategies to contain meditation into your each day routine.

Morning rituals

Start the day with a quick meditation. Sit in a quiet place, breathe deeply, and focus on the present second. This creates a first-rate foundation for the day and promotes inner peace.

Mindful breathing:

Incorporate aware respiratory into your each day life. Whether you're taking walks, eating, or jogging, focus on your respiration. This is the way you create a aware smash to your annoying regular existence.

Lunch spoil for meditation:

Use your lunch break to do a quick meditation. Find a quiet place, close your eyes and consciousness to your respiratory. Just 5 mins can help reduce pressure and recharge your batteries.

Meditate at Work:

Create a small meditation region at paintings. Take small breaks and deal with your mind.

Your mental clarity and productivity will enhance.

Relaxation within the night:

Make it a dependancy to meditate within the night time to give up the day consciously. Think approximately the day's events and forget about approximately them. This calms the mind and promotes restful sleep.

Mindfulness in every day existence:

Practice mindfulness in everyday existence. Whether you are washing dishes, showering, or cooking, interest on the prevailing 2nd. This promotes a conscious life.

Technology withdrawal:

Schedule a technology detox frequently. Consciously flip off your telephone or unique gadgets for a while. Dedicate this time to quiet meditation and experiencing nature.

Group meditation:

Join a close-by meditation organization or start your private meditation employer. Meditating together creates a collegial environment and promotes shared reports.

Meditation in advance than mattress:

At the give up of the day, do a calming meditation. Practice breathing sports and guided meditations to lighten up the mind and promote restful sleep.

Mindfulness in relationships:

Integrate mindfulness into interpersonal relationships. Listen actively, be present and be affected character. Mindfulness promotes deeper connections and improves the quality of relationships.

Daily reflected photo:

Take a quick time for reflected photo each day. Ask yourself how you have protected meditation into your every day life, what issues you've got triumph over, and what awesome adjustments you have got noticed.

Incorporating meditation into normal lifestyles requires continuity and mindfulness. By consciously making use of those techniques to severa elements of everyday lifestyles, you could experience the transformative electricity of meditation and integrate it sustainably into your properly-being.

Chapter 9: The Importance of Ritual in Tarot Meditation

The significance of rituals in Tarot meditation is profound in that they create a structured and symbolic environment that enriches the non secular journey. This chapter examines in element the feature of formality in tarot meditation. From developing a sacred area to integrating the ritual into card studying, it gives sensible guidance on the manner to correctly combine the ritual into your meditation exercise.

Create a sacred area

It is essential to set up a sacred place for tarot meditation. Choose a quiet vicinity in which there are not any distractions. Energetically cleanse this place the usage of incense, crystals, or prayers. This manner you create an energetically amazing surroundings appropriate for non secular paintings.

Meaning of the symbols:

Use symbols in sacred space to create a deeper connection with tarot meditation. Place symbols that have non-public which means, together with tarot playing gambling playing cards, candles, or stones. These symbols can function a bridge the various bodily international and the non secular aircraft.

Include factors.

Include elements consisting of earth, water, fireside and air for your rituals. Use appropriate props or symbolic representations of the factors in a sacred area. This promotes harmony with the forces of nature and deepens your connection to non secular practices.

The Importance of Time and Seasons:

When growing rituals, undergo in thoughts time and seasons. Use the energy cycles of the day and yr to guide your meditation. For instance, the levels of the moon or the summer season solstice can provide time to focus on a selected query or problem in a tarot meditation.

Include exercising:

Incorporate conscious motion into your rituals. These may be dances, mild yoga sporting sports or arm waving. Incorporating movement releases energy inside the body and creates a dynamic connection to tarot meditation.

Ritualized respiration sports:

The mixture of respiration sporting activities and rituals creates a deeper connection to meditation. The hobby is on conscious breathing, deep belly respiration and rhythmic respiration patterns. This no longer first-class allows rest but moreover allows non secular exercising.

The Power of Repetition:

Rituals benefit their strength through repetition. Create a solid regular which you regularly incorporate into your Tarot meditation. This can be lights a candle, shuffling the playing gambling playing cards, or saying a unique affirmation. Repetitions beautify the lively resonance of the ritual.

Klangintegration:

Use gadgets which include creating a track bowls, drums or rattles to characteristic an acoustic dimension to the ritual. Sounds can create a special atmosphere and harmonize the vibrations within the room. Experiment with particular sounds to find out the best that is maximum effective for you.

The Importance of Intention.

Set a smooth purpose in your ritual. Before you begin a tarot meditation, you ought to take into account what goals you need to reap. Set a smooth motive and move into the ritual with emotional power. A smooth cause serves as a manual for the strength that builds all through meditation.

Integrate the ritual into card reading:

Seamlessly be a part of the ritual with the cardboard reading technique. Before reading the playing cards, carry out a brief ritual to pay interest. Shuffle the playing cards, recite affirmations or invoke specific energies. Incorporating rituals deepens the connection with you, the playing cards and the non secular region.

Care of formality equipment:

Treat ritual items with understand and care. Cleanse and energize it often. This ensures the effectiveness of the ritual and strengthens your connection to it.

Reflection after the ritual.

At the prevent of every ritual, do a quick mirrored image. Write down your stories, emotions and observations in a ritual magazine. In this way, you may benefit a deeper data of your spiritual direction and be capable of music its improvement over time.

The ritual in Tarot meditation gives a based totally framework for deepening your spiritual experience. Consciously incorporating symbols, elements, movement, respiratory techniques, and easy intentions into rituals can beautify the transformative strength of tarot meditation and create a deeper reference to the religious global.

Dealing with Emotions during Meditation

Dealing with feelings at some point of meditation is both an crucial mission and a key to deeper knowledge. This bankruptcy takes a better have a take a look at the complicated connections among emotions throughout meditation. From identification and popularity to focused emotion law, it offers practical commands and insights that make it less difficult to cope with emotions in a healthful manner in meditation workout.

The nature of feelings

Understand the essential nature of feelings. Emotions are natural reactions to internal or out of doors stimuli and mirror our modern-day emotional united states of america.

Emotions are part of the human enjoy and can be felt extra intensely in the course of meditation.

Develop mindfulness of emotions:

Develop mindfulness of feelings. Observe with an unbiased and open attitude. Allow emotions to waft throughout mindfulness respiratory and splendid meditations.

Recognize feelings:

Learn to discover emotions. Associate the phrases with the feelings professional in the course of meditation. This allows for additonal correct self-reflected photo and permits the device of emotion law.

Accepting emotions:

Practice accepting emotions. Don't fight the emotion, gain it as part of the existing second. Acceptance allows you to experience feelings with out resistance and promotes inner peace.

The feature of thoughts:

Become aware about the relationship among feelings and mind. Emotions are often observed through mind. Observe what idea patterns emerge in some unspecified time inside the destiny of sure feelings. This will assist you higher recognize the underlying beliefs.

Emotion regulation techniques:

Learn one of a type emotion law strategies. Breathing physical video video games, contemporary muscle relaxation, and mindfulness carrying sports can assist lessen emotional depth. Try special strategies to discover the simplest that works first-class for you.

Conscious hobby:

When disturbing feelings get up, consciously recognition your interest on your respiration or a few other meditation. This allows you to look at the emotion with out being overwhelmed with the aid of it. Conscious interest creates distance among you and the feeling.

Let bypass of control:

Practice letting skip of manipulate. Emotions regularly rise up at a deeper level of consciousness and cannot typically be controlled rationally. Letting move of manage may not imply suppressing the feelings, however instead looking at and permitting them.

Physical notion of feelings:

Pay interest to the bodily sensations related to the emotions. For instance, tension, tension, disenchanted stomach, and so on. Observe those sensations and allow them to get up with out resistance.

Creative expression of feelings:

Consider expressing feelings creatively. Express your emotions by using way of the usage of writing an emotional journal, drawing, or dancing. Creative expression allows for deeper processing and release of emotional strength.

Mindful self-mirrored photograph:

After meditation, take time for aware self-reflected picture. Ask your self what feelings arose, the way you treated them, and what insights you obtained approximately your inner self. Self-reflected picture promotes personal growth and information.

Seek expert aid:

If sure emotions are very sturdy or stand up regularly, you have to no longer hesitate to searching for professional manual. An experienced therapist can assist and manual you in processing your emotions greater deeply all through meditation. Working with emotions throughout meditation is a profound workout that requires mindfulness, popularity, and targeted emotional manipulate.

Chapter 10: Developing Intuition through Tarot Meditation

Developing intuition through Tarot meditation is an attractive way to strengthen your non secular powers. This financial ruin takes a better check the mechanics of instinct and offers sensible guidance at the manner to include Tarot meditation into the development of intuition. From sprucing your senses to decoding tarot playing cards as an intuitive device, this financial ruin offers in-depth insights into developing your intuitive skills.

Understanding intuition

Start with a easy information of intuition. Intuition is the ability to recognize records proper away and non-analytically. It is a herbal part of human notion and can be strengthened through conscious practice.

Attention to internal indicators

Develop mindfulness for inner indicators. Pay interest to subtle emotions, intuitions, and pictures that upward thrust up at some point of tarot meditation. These internal signs provide clues for intuitive insights.

Connecting with the Tarot gambling playing cards

Strengthen your connection to the tarot gambling playing playing cards. Consider the tarot gambling cards now not handiest as a fortune-telling device, however moreover as a gateway to a deeper diploma of attention. Deepen your relationship with the symbols and energies of the playing cards.

Strengthen your senses:

Strengthen your senses through mindfulness wearing activities. During tarot meditation, consciously cognizance on the senses: sight, paying attention to, contact, perfume and taste. Sharpening the senses opens the door to extra intuition.

The because of this that of desires:

Pay interest to goals as a supply of intuitive facts. Dreams are a powerful medium for intuitive messages. Keep a dream magazine and undergo in thoughts the symbolism to your dreams.

The role of meditation strategies:

Use specific meditation techniques to deepen your intuitive popularity. During meditation, interest your hobby at the zero.33 eye or coronary coronary heart area. This attention opens energetic channels for intuitive insights.

Practical bodily video games for intuitive perception:

Incorporate sensible sports activities into your tarot meditation. Intuitively draw gambling cards and have a observe what feelings and mind arise. Let your intuition guide you and delve deeper into the which means of the gambling playing cards.

The Importance of Trust:

Have self perception for your intuitive abilities. Don't doubt the intuitions and messages that upward thrust up for the duration of a tarot meditation. Trust strengthens your connection to internal recognition.

Handle doubts carefully:

Be careful whilst dealing with doubts and skepticism. Doubt is part of religious boom. Accept him, but do now not allow him get the pinnacle hand. When you receive doubts, you could deal with them consciously.

Connection with nature:

To beef up your instinct, are trying to find a reference to nature. Spend time outside, meditating underneath a tree or looking on the sky. Nature is a supply of strength and facts that could help the development of your instinct.

The Role of Compassion:

Develop compassion for your self and others. Intuition is associated with an open coronary coronary heart. Compassion creates an environment of receptivity that promotes intuitive notion.

Incorporate intuition into every day life

Consciously combine instinct into your ordinary existence. Choose to pay interest to your instinct in everyday situations. Watch how your options and movements trade.

Reflection and further improvement

Reflect frequently at the improvement of your instinct. Keep a magazine of what improvement you have located, what stressful conditions have arisen, and what insights have emerged on your tarot meditations. Introspection promotes non-stop increase.

Developing your intuitive capabilities via Tarot meditation is an exciting adventure that gives each religious intensity and practical utility. By integrating the ideas and practices supplied here, you could open yourself to a deeper reference to the intuitive data that lies inner you.

Chapter 11: What Exactly Is Meditation?

Meditation is the deliberate workout of spending time with our minds. We take day journey of our annoying days to sit down, breathe, and cope with our respiratory. This assists us in turning into extra privy to our mind, appearing more compassionately within the route of ourselves and others, and connecting with the prevailing 2nd.

People may also equate meditation with sitting in quiet and ceasing all mind and feelings to be able to emerge as peaceful. However, that isn't how the thoughts works, and neither does meditation we education letting mind come and go rather than looking to forestall them.

How can we accomplish this? Consider ideas to be like internet site on-line traffic in the mind, always speeding with the resource of.

When we get caught up in analyzing or assessing a belief or turning into misplaced in a fable, we may additionally have a look at a shiny automobile and rush after it. Sometimes we enjoy an obstacle earlier and try to avoid it, definitely as we do at the same time as we assume or enjoy anything unsightly. Meditation teaches us to observe internet page traffic without chasing or combating it, in reality permitting the idea to come returned lower back and bypass. Then, to permit the idea bypass, gently switch our hobby far away from it and again onto our breath.

The greater we guidance, the extra we can be able to recognize ideas for what they will be: actually thoughts. It turns into a lot much less complicated to allow subjects cross and "get out of our heads" an outstanding way to be extra immersed in what we're doing, whether or now not or no longer it is spending time with own family, self-care, or going for walks in competition to a reduce-off date.

What is the purpose of meditation?

Life may be unpleasant, annoying, and hard at instances. We have no manipulate over what takes area, however we do have the functionality to steer how we react to it. To apprehend our very personal thoughts (our thoughts, emotions, and behaviours), we need to be conscious. And we require compassion that allows you to connect with ourselves and others.

No rely what goes on in our existence, meditation allows us to peer topics more without a doubt, experience calmer and happier, and be kind to ourselves and others. However, this doesn't guarantee that we are capable of revel in smooth, calm, and compassionate as fast as we start or surrender. Because the thoughts are continuously evolving, our experience can also regulate each time we meditate.

We're coaching ourselves to be content material cloth with our minds as they may be. It in reality is that clean. Meditation isn't approximately performing some element aside from training it: slowing down at some stage in our traumatic days, checking in with ourselves, and seeing how our minds are because meditation is all approximately being kind with our minds.

What do I want to get started out with meditation?

Meditation does now not want a good deal effort. However, knowing the following meditation basics makes it less difficult to begin started:

What is maximum critical is consistency.

We ought to meditate commonly in keeping with week, if no longer every day. However, even definitely one meditation can reason a discount in thoughts wandering. The more we guidance, the extra blessings we are able to enjoy. According to investigate, 30 days of Headspace decreases strain by one-1/3 and increases life pleasure.

Meditation classes, like exercise training or appointments, can be beneficial to set up. We also can embody it into an present habitual, together with while we shower or easy our tooth.

It's awesome if we skip an afternoon or . We can also furthermore certainly resume from wherein we left off.

The pinnacle-excellent time to meditate is every time we have got the possibility.

It makes no difference whilst (or in which) we meditate, so pick out out something time works excellent for you. Meditation might be useful to exercising first trouble inside the morning in advance than beginning our day, or at night time earlier than going to bed. We should usually meditate in advance than our final corporation assembly or after losing the kids off at faculty. Instead of pushing through whilst we are beaten, we'd take a pause and meditate.

Meditation in reality takes a couple of minutes.

A 5-minute meditation is sufficient. If that isn't sufficient, a ten-minute meditation is good for novices. We can also regularly increase our time if we've a steady exercise.

Be organized for distracting noises.

We don't need complete silence to meditate. For novices, common quiet in meditation may be too daunting. When everything is silent, we grow to be hypersensitive to any noise.

In any case, life isn't always regularly tranquil. We may additionally anticipate disturbances in our meditation workout, whether or not it's loud track from a neighbour, a domestic dog barking in the street, a truck backing up or sounds in some distinctive room at domestic. Instead of being disillusioned and targeted on the noise, "Why is my neighbour having a dance celebration proper now?" or trying to shut it out, "I want this song may forestall," we can also moreover study our thinking, let it circulate, and pass back to our breath.

We can continuously use earplugs, noise-cancelling headphones, white noise turbines, or exciting tune, which encompass the Focus track inside the Headspace app, to assist us pay interest.

Sit and get dressed whichever you want.

We can take a seat down everywhere we love at some point of the meditation so long as our decrease again is straight away, our neck and shoulders are comfortable, and our chin is lightly tucked. We can sit on our couch, a eating or place of work chair, or on a cushion propped up thru cushions at the mattress. Cross or uncross your arms and legs as seems herbal. Consider enjoyable any clothes this is too tight, commencing our shoes, or putting off any item that reasons us to fidget.

To studies from experts, attempt guided meditation.

Guided meditation is a form of meditation in which an trainer instructs you on what to do. They train us on even as to open and close to our eyes, the manner to breathe, and exclusive meditation practices. They provide first-rate belief and practical propose to novices, which consist of guidelines for applying what we examine within the direction of meditation in actual lifestyles, due to the fact they'll be specialists on how the mind operates.

Once we're comfortable with the technique, we are able to try unguided meditation on our personal.

There is not any accurate or incorrect method to meditate.

It's proper if we have were given trouble meditating on the begin It happens to everyone. Even if we're wondering if we're meditating successfully, don't forget that those are simplest thoughts.

Chapter 12: What Takes Location While You Meditate?

What takes place if we "do not anything" in the course of meditation? Here's what you may count on:

Our thoughts will wander. Even specialists are sidetracked by means of the use of thoughts within the course of meditation and forget to comply with their breath, because the mind will constantly suppose irrespective of how masses we schooling.

So, what must I do? Return our attention from our distracted thoughts to our breath. This educates the thoughts to be more quite simply distracted. We'll in the end find out that we can meditate for prolonged durations of time with out being distracted.

We won't enjoy whatever. This does now not imply that we're doing some component incorrectly or that we ought to surrender.

So, what must I do? Instead of allowing uncertainty to paralyse us, we need to take it each day and constantly checking in. When we meditate, we also can remind ourselves that we aren't dropping time. We're searching after our minds.

We can be moved to tears. Maybe we're impatient, indignant, bored, or livid at some point of one exercising, then involved, traumatic, or depressed the following. Because the thoughts is so used to being busy, it's natural for all of our emotions and tension to floor even as we ultimately loosen up.

So, what want to I do? Trying to push feelings away will absolutely cause them to greater acute. Allow them the gap they require, then permit them to go. It may be beneficial to be aware of how emotions sense within the frame. Is it worry that motives us to tighten our fists? Is tension making us sweat? Is it boredom that reasons us to area out? Then we may try to relieve a number of that tension the use of the breath.

We'll be antsy. When we strive to sit down motionless, whether or not or not at some point of meditation or otherwise, we're capable of't assist however scratch an itch, make bigger our neck, or pass and uncross our legs.

So, what must I do? We can also deal with this traditional sensation within the same way we technique distracting thoughts: find out at the identical time as we're fidgeting, permit it circulate, and repair our attention to our breath.

We'll maximum likely try too difficult. Meditating is not just like gaining new abilties. The greater paintings we positioned into maximum subjects, the more we reap out of them. However, meditation is more much like sleep. The tougher we strive to sleep, the more hard it's miles to fall asleep. When we take a seat right down to meditation, despite the fact that we try very difficult to clean our minds, they generally generally generally tend to experience whole.

So, what want to I do?

There isn't such a element as the right meditation. If we see ourselves becoming dissatisfied due to the reality the visitors in our minds is flowing too fast, or if we question, "Why is this so tough?" we may moreover moreover show ourselves a few compassion. Let out a deep sigh to supply our interest lower again to the breath.

We is probably tired. Don't fear if we go to sleep. The thoughts is becoming aware of distinguishing among slowing down and shutting down.

So, what want to I do? Try sitting instead of lying down to keep your thoughts attentive.

Mindfulness for Beginners: What It Is & How to Practice

Mindfulness is interest of the prevailing 2nd.1 Beginners and experts alike can exercise techniques to live attentive and attuned to their environments. Beginner mindfulness wearing events can encompass conscious ingesting, walking, or deep breathing.

What Is Mindfulness?

At its center, mindfulness is a dating with your self and the arena spherical you. Mindfulness is clean as it isn't a few exclusive set of policies and thoughts to memorize. It's not a flashy fad with hollow ensures of a notable life or a brief-repair method to happiness. Instead, mindfulness is a way of existence and concerning your self, others, and situations lightly and purposefully, regardless of what obstacles, stressors, and stressful situations pop into your path.

Mindfulness lets in you to live for your real moments in preference to be trapped for your thoughts and emotions approximately the beyond, gift, or future—your mind is full of the tangible elements of the prevailing second that you take in together together together with your senses. You stay at face fee rather than implementing judgments or expectations on yourself or your reports.2

Mindfulness consists of paying hobby and noticing in that you are, who you're with, and what you're doing.3

People often surprise whether or not or no longer or no longer mindfulness is a religious manner of life. While it's far important for Hinduism, Buddhism, Judaism, Christianity, and Islam, mindfulness moreover exists independently of spirituality.Four Everyone can feature their very personal meaning to their practice and life because of the reality mindfulness is a courting and approach to dwelling with out set tips and rituals.

Key Concepts of Mindfulness for Beginners

Mindfulness overrides the thoughts and body's computerized response to our conditions, thoughts, and emotions. Using deep respiratory and your senses (sight, sound, touch, fragrance, and taste) to pay interest at the winning 2nd decreases interest to your sympathetic nervous device (the only chargeable for the combat-or-flight stress response) and activates your parasympathetic involved device (the relaxation-and-digest calm response).Five,6,7

However, mindfulness does now not give up right proper right here. Mindfulness tool will let you calm your mind as fast as you have got were given taken charge of your frame and moved a ways out of your stress reaction.

Mindfulness includes those underlying elements:4,7,eight

Breathing

People who exercise yogic breathing use the Sanskrit term pranayama or controlled breathing. Working together along with your breath to alternate from shallow, short breaths to gradual, deep breaths sets the foundation for mindfulness. In aware respiration, you popularity at the sound and experience of air getting into and leaving your body to refocus bad mind and calm your body.

Observation & Awareness

When you interest on the winning 2d, you take it in alongside aspect your senses and grow to be extra aware of your self, others, and every state of affairs. You can decide what to do at the equal time as you're conscious, even of terrible emotions or annoying sports. You can't see what you have to do to trouble-remedy even as caught for your thoughts, juggling and tripping over your thoughts and feelings. By tuning in virtually to what's happening proper now, you are extra aware on your lifestyles.

Nonjudgmental Acceptance & Openness

Of course, you don't want to love every experience. However, you moreover mght don't need to fight in opposition to them. When we conflict and withstand our thoughts or conditions, we stay centered on the awful. The more we judge topics, the extra effective they come to be due to the fact that's wherein our attention lies. In mindfulness, you note some aspect and take transport of it for what it's far. You also are open to your memories as they come. Then, you could embody what is going properly and each permit skip of what's bothering you or determine to take useful moves to alternate it.

Intentional Focus

Mindfulness allows you to select out your cognizance in preference to having your awful thoughts, emotions, and conditions devour your interest and energy. Every time you song in to sensations within the present 2d, you pay interest on cause to the people you're with and the things you are doing. If you're ingesting ice cream along facet your youngsters or a friend, as an instance, in desire to missing the enjoy due to the truth you're misplaced in idea, you reflect onconsideration on factors of the instant and the revel in of being with a person you revel in.

What Is the Goal of Mindfulness?

Mindfulness permits beginners and professionals alike to live in the gift 2d, one 2d at a time. The goal of mindfulness is calming poor mind and feelings so that you can pick your moves. Living mindfully permits you to take decrease once more your existence from the boundaries retaining you trapped and stay in step with your values (due to the fact your existence does depend).Nine

Mindfulness isn't a magic wand with the intention to put off troubles and disturbing situations. Instead, it permits you to increase calm, impartial recognition of your mind, feelings, physical sensations, and behaviors.10 Mindfulness allows you damage unfastened out of your problems and continue to be calm and focused so you can reply to issues with intention in vicinity of reacting emotionally.2

How to Practice Mindfulness for Beginners

One of the first-rate topics about mindfulness is that it's also to be had. You don't need to spend coins or buy precise system. All mindfulness calls for is your self—a few factor you constantly have with you. Further, you can exercise mindfulness precisely how you're. You don't need to take education or do a little element to prepare for it.

Mindfulness for beginners can be formal and informal.7,9 Many people use a combination of the 2. A formal mindfulness practice consists of placing aside time daily to interact in mindfulness wearing activities. When you devote time to recognize, you develop your functionality to maintain your hobby for an extended length.

Informal mindfulness is mindfulness on the bypass. You flip your hobby to a few aspect inside the present 2d, anywhere you're and some aspect you're doing. For example, you could feel anxious and annoyed at the same time as dashing to an appointment. Rather than stewing at a crimson slight, watch the motors going via the intersection the other way and observe records about them.

You can also use mindfulness informally at some stage in fantastic conditions to make the most out of them. For instance, if you're gambling together with your children, pull your hobby to the triumphing second with the resource of being attentive to their laughter.

Mindfulness Techniques for Beginners

Mindfulness is a manner of being with your self and your global and a skills you could develop. The concept is to do each mindfulness technique together along with your full attention. Remember the precept of non-judgment at the same time as your thoughts wanders (and it probably will). Don't become irritated with yourself due to the fact your attention wanders. Simply look at your thoughts and skip again your interest to the hobby.

Below are seven hints on mindfulness for beginners:

1. Focused Breathing

Whenever you've got a have a look at your self turning into careworn, pause in which you're and close to your eyes in case you enjoy comfortable doing so. Place your fingers to your belly and enjoy your body upward thrust and fall as you breathe. Inhale slowly thru your nose and reputation at the sound and experience of the air getting into your frame. Fill your lungs in order that your stomach expands. Pause for a few seconds. Exhale slowly and in reality, yet again taking note of the sound and enjoy of the air leaving your body.

You may also choice to strive the kind of variations:

When you inhale, say a word or word to your self. You can also say, "In breath." When you exhale, mentally repeat a particular phrase or phrase like, "Out breath." You can also use phrases like "calm," "peace," "joy," "presence," or every other phrase that is extensive and motivating for you.

Count as you breathe. See how long you can make every inhale and exhale—six seconds? Eight? Twelve? You can try and maintain your in-breaths and out-breaths equal or make your exhale slightly longer.

2. Simply Notice

Close your eyes. Take one or extra aware breaths. Open your eyes and soak up what's round you. What do you notice? What sounds do you concentrate? Is there a crucial scent? What textures do you experience? Just phrase with out getting stuck thinking about some component especially.

Use the opportunity to growth a mindfulness precept known as coming unhooked.Eleven Too regularly, we become hooked through issues. We emerge as stuck on them as we consider them again and again. In mindfulness, you may note your hooks and allow them to be there with out judging or struggling. Notice your hook and then extend your awareness to one-of-a-kind subjects round you. You slip off the hook and into your existence in that 2nd at the identical time as you be aware of the super topics spherical you.

3. Take a Mindful Walk

Take a damage from a stressful scenario and engage your mind and body with a mindful stroll. You can do this outside or inner. If you may, do away with your socks and footwear to sense your feet shifting at the ground or ground (but if this isn't sensible, that's adequate. You can mindfully stroll together collectively together with your shoes on). Begin to stroll at your very personal tempo. It's regularly advocated to stroll slowly. However, you can set your tempo if this feels uncomfortable.

Focus in your feet, feeling them connect to the ground as you bypass. Next, popularity in your frame. How do your muscular tissues and joints go along with the waft? How is your posture? Notice the nuances of your frame in movement. Then, turn your attention to what's round you. What is the temperature? Is there wind blowing air at some stage in your pores and pores and skin? What are you capable of contact to enjoy special textures? What sounds do you pick out up? What do you note? Walk mindfully as long as you are able.

four. Have a Mindful Snack or Meal

Mindful eating is a healthy experience that calms the thoughts and body for correct digestion. Many people will be predisposed to devour in a hurry, gulping our food brief amongst sports. Other times, we're distracted on the equal time as we devour, poking spherical on our telephones or looking tv.

Hone your mindfulness talents and nurture your self by manner of the use of consuming mindfully. Pay interest to what you're doing as you prepare your meals, relishing within the textures and scents. Then, fully experience your food as you devour. Sit and not using a problem and grow to be aware about your posture. Let your self revel in the flavor of the food and enjoy of ingesting.

5. Do a Body Scan

When you're careworn, take a moment to check in along side your body. You can lie down, sit down down down, or stand. Close your eyes if possible. Starting at your ft and taking walks bit by bit up to your face and head, attend to each location of your body. Do you be aware your self preserving tension everywhere? If so, hold your focus in that spot a bit longer. Take a sluggish, deep breath, and remember the healthy oxygen flowing proper to the stressful spot to assist it relax. The more you check in together with your frame, the higher you may prevent it from defensive stress and anxiety.

6. Listen to Music

The subsequent time you pay interest in your preferred track, do it mindfully. Give the experience your complete interest. Can you pick out out unique gadgets? Pay hobby to the voice of the singer, if there can be one. Immerse your self completely in the sounds in choice to letting them run within the history on the equal time as you recall different things.

7. Center Yourself

When pressured or in any other case emotional, you can use this clean mindfulness technique to relax out and loosen up. Place the hands of your arms flat on any floor (a tabletop, your legs, or a few trouble else that is accessible). Concentrate at the manner it feels to your fingertips, down the duration of your hands, and in the route of your palms. As you acquire this, start to take numerous gradual, deep breaths.

How Does Mindfulness Help?

Mindfulness lets in you be completely present for the pleased moments and remain calm sooner or later of stressful ones. You learn how to approach lifestyles with openness and curiosity in vicinity of judgment, helping reduce anxiety and increase a feel of reason and which means.10 Intentionally shifting your popularity adjustments how your brain responds to pressure and systems inside the mind. As referred to, mindfulness doesn't make issues disappear but changes the manner you manage those issues.

Improvements related to mindfulness encompass:[2,10,12]

Reduced anxiety signs and symptoms

Reduced melancholy

Improved submit-stressful pressure ailment (PTSD)

Decreased dating, artwork, and distinct life pressure

Existential problems and problems related to lifestyles transitions

Increased nicely-being

Improved conduct law

Reduced strain associated with persistent pain

Boosted immune machine functioning

Increased hobby span and consciousness

Improved empathy and tolerance

Heightened resilience

Mindfulness for Beginners Examples

The electricity of mindfulness is seemingly endless. People of every age and backgrounds can use it throughout all situations to live calm notwithstanding challenges and live clearly in every 2d, addressing issues thoughtfully and embracing high quality critiques.

Mindfulness for ADHD

Mindfulness for beginners with ADHD may additionally additionally growth awareness and popularity.Thirteen The beauty of mindfulness is that it wishes neither strict techniques nor a minimum quantity of time. Someone with ADHD can start training mindfulness little by little, that specialize in their breath for one minute (or maybe only some breaths) or taking a aware walk to the surrender of their driveway.

Even short mindfulness physical activities can growth the ability to self-adjust and pay interest for prolonged intervals. Focusing on the instantaneous and cultivating an open and accepting mindset permits human beings with ADHD assume without a doubt and gently. They can look for styles in their behavior and make small modifications that result in massive upgrades in their lives.

Mindfulness for Depression

Studies show that packages the usage of mindfulness, including mindfulness-primarily based cognitive remedy (MBCT), can be as powerful as antidepressants in preventing melancholy relapse.14 Mindfulness gives people control over their thoughts, allowing them to understand their awful thoughts and purposefully attention instead on the excellent factors of the existing second. As people expand new views, their symptoms of depression fade and are an awful lot less probable to go again.

Mindfulness During Stressful Situations

Practicing mindfulness can help humans cope certainly with strain. As visible, mindfulness impacts extraordinary modifications within the mind and body, assisting flip off the fight-or-flight response and prompt the calming relaxation-and-digest reaction. As we discover ways to stay focused on the present second, we beautify our potential to deal surely with stressors as an alternative of getting stuck up in horrific thoughts and emotions about them.15

Mindfulness lets in us emerge as aware about our emotions and awful reactions so we will shift to extra beneficial behaviors, changing our perception of strain to stay calm and targeted.Sixteen

Benefits of Mindfulness for Beginners

Mindfulness improves each our physiological (body-based totally) and highbrow (concept-

and emotion-targeted) responses to problems and demanding situations. We can acquire top notch advantages as we decorate our ability to stay focused at the winning 2nd and revel in it nonjudgmentally.

Living mindfully can lower stress, anxiety, despair, perceptions of pain, and immoderate blood pressure. Further, it may decorate awareness, sleep, or even ailment manage, which includes better control of diabetes.Nine

Mindfulness gives awesome benefits, too. As you learn how to be present and open, you increase greater self-reputation and a extra balanced angle on lifestyles, accepting what you may't alternate, taking intentional movement to trade what you may, and that specialize in what is right in region of what is inaccurate.7

Is Mindfulness for Beginners Effective?

Researchers preserve to behavior research to analyze the effectiveness of mindfulness. One have a observe positioned that human beings conscious with the resource of nature revel in decrease tension and react a whole lot less emotionally within the face of issues.17 Further research shows that mindfulness interventions extensively reduce despair signs and symptoms and signs and symptoms and symptoms.18 Thus, many wonderful research file comparable conclusions: mindfulness is powerful in assisting people show up for their lives and respond thoughtfully to problems and stressors.

Final Thoughts

The most effective manner to begin residing mindfully is to clearly start. Catch your poor thoughts and feelings earlier than refocusing your interest on the present. Be open to your evaluations without judging or suffering closer to them so that you can stay calm and reply thoughtfully and positively. As with some element, exercise makes first-rate. The greater you exercise mindfulness strategies for novices, the greater natural mindfulness becomes.

Chapter 13: Learn the Art and Basic Techniques with These Pointers

Meditation is a few factors that everybody can exercise at any time, from everywhere – even in noisy surroundings. It's easy to analyze and employs some vital strategies. The greater we meditate, the greater comfortable we can get with spending time with our minds.

It doesn't take lengthy to be conscious the blessings of everyday meditation exercise. According to investigate, Headspace can lower strain in as low as 10 days. Thousands of studies have additionally confirmed that mindfulness and meditation can also additionally decorate each highbrow and bodily health. So, regardless of why we need to begin meditating — to enjoy tons much less forced, sleep better, be extra centered, or enhance relationships — each meditation brings us one step inside the direction of growing healthful conduct for a happy mind.

Meditation is the most essential addiction I've advanced in the very last ten years of addiction formation. Without a doubt, hands down.

Meditation has helped me installation all of my other behavior; it has helped me come to be more tranquil, focused, much less worried with ache, and extra thankful and touchy to the entirety in my life. I'm some distance from best, however it's gotten me an extended manner.

Most drastically, it has assisted me in understanding my very very own psyche. I never notion approximately what grow to be taking location inner my thoughts until I commenced out meditating; it virtually happened, and I discovered its guidelines like an automaton. All of that still takes place nowadays, but I'm turning into extra aware about what's taking area. I can also additionally select out whether or not or not or no longer to obey the orders. I understand myself higher (now not absolutely), which has boosted my flexibility and freedom.

So ... This is a workout I strongly recommend. And, at the same time as I'm now not claiming it's clean, you could start small and decorate as you education. Don't anticipate to be accurate proper away - that's why they name it "exercising"!

These recommendations aren't intended to help you turn out to be an expert; as an alternative, they have to help you get started and preserve going. You don't ought to try them unexpectedly; try a pair, return to this newsletter, and strive one or more.

Sit for no more than minutes. It will appear stupidly clean to meditate for 2 minutes. That is remarkable. Begin with minutes every day for every week. If it's miles going properly, add some other minutes and repeat for in step with week. If the whole thing is going as deliberate, you'll be meditating for 10 mins every day thru the second one month, that is extremely good! But first, start small.

Do it first issue within the morning every day. It's smooth to mention, "I'll meditate each day," however then fail to comply with via. Instead, set a reminder for each morning whilst you stand up, and depart a "mediate" phrase anyplace you'll be aware it.

Don't get bogged down with the how; just do it. Most people are concerned with wherein to take a seat, the manner to take a seat down, what cushion to use… all of that is first-rate, however it isn't crucial to get commenced out. Begin through genuinely sitting in a chair or for your sofa. Or even on your bed. Sit cross-legged in case you're cushty at the floor. It'll virtually be for 2 minutes earlier than the entirety, so simply sit down down. Later, you could fear about optimising it so you may be comfortable for longer durations of time, but for now, virtually take a seat down somewhere quiet and cushty.

Check in to look the way you're doing. Simply take a look at in with yourself to evaluate the manner you're feeling as you start your meditation workout. How do you experience in your frame? How is the kingdom of your thoughts? Busy? Tired? Anxious? Accept a few trouble you supply to this meditation consultation as really OK.

Take a few deep breaths. Now which you've settled in, attention on your breathing. Simply attention your hobby in your inhalation and comply with it thru your nose all the way in your lungs. Count "one" as you're taking your first breath in, then "" as you exhale. Repeat until the count number of ten, then start yet again at one.

Come flow once more if you get lost. Your thoughts will wander. This is nearly really authentic.

There is not any difficulty with that. When your thoughts wanders, simply smile and softly circulate back on your breath. Recount "one" and start yet again. You may additionally need to revel in annoyed, but it's honestly ordinary to lose attention; absolutely everyone do. This is exercising, and also you won't be very good at it for a time.

Create a loving attitude. When you spot mind and emotions rise up for the duration of meditation, technique them with a kind mindset. Consider them pals in desire to intruders or adversaries. They are a part of you, however not the entire you. Be pleasant in desire to impolite.

Don't be too worried about doing subjects wrong. You'll be concerned that you're doing it incorrectly. That's OK; every body do. You're not performing some detail incorrectly. There is not any first rate manner to carry out it; sincerely be grateful which you are doing it.

Don't be worried approximately cleansing your head. Many people take shipping of as real with that meditation is prepared cleaning your thoughts or preventing all mind. It isn't. This does take vicinity sometimes, but it is not the "goal" of meditation. It's herbal to have mind. We're all accountable of it. Our brains are thinking factories that we cannot just flip off. Instead, clearly training focussing your interest and repeat at the same time as your thoughts wanders.

Stay with a few aspect comes up. When mind or sensations arise, and they may, attempt to live with them for a time. Yes, I understand I advocated to go back to the breath, however after consistent with week of exercise, you could strive sticking with an arising concept or sensation. We try and keep away from sensations like annoyance, wrath, and worry... however staying with the enjoy for an prolonged is a completely precious meditation exercising. Simply live and be intrigued.

Learn approximately your self. This approach is ready analyzing how your thoughts works, no longer just focusing your attention. What precisely goes on interior? It's hazy, however via manner of seeing how your mind wanders, will become annoyed, avoids hard thoughts... you may begin to recognize your self.

Make new friends with your self. Learn approximately oneself with a kind thoughts-set in preference to a crucial one. You're mastering a cutting-edge acquaintance. Give yourself a grin and a few self-love.

Perform a body take a look at. You may also moreover consciousness your attention on one frame location at a time after you've gotten a chunk higher at following your breath. Begin collectively together with your ft's soles - how do they experience? Move slowly in your toes, hints of your feet, ankles, and all the way to the pinnacle of your head.

Take be aware about the mild, noises, and electricity. After you've practiced together in conjunction with your breath for at the least each week, a few different area to interest your hobby is the slight all round you. Simply fix your gaze on one component and take within the mild in the room. Another day, really be aware of noises. Try to take a look at the energy inside the room all round you (in conjunction with mild and noises) each different day.

Make a enterprise commitment. Don't simply reply, "Sure, I'll try this for more than one days." Make a agency determination to this. Be devoted for your mind for at least a month.

It is viable to do it wherever. You can meditate on your place of business if you're traveling or if some thing comes up within the morning. In a park. During your journey. While strolling someplace. Sitting meditation is the greatest location to begin, but in truth, you're running toward mindfulness all of the time.

Continue with the guided meditation. To start, you can strive following guided meditations if it allows. Tara Brach's guided meditations are pretty useful to my spouse.

Check in together collectively along with your pals. While I want to meditate on my own, you can accomplish that together together with your partner, kid, or buddy. Or honestly do not forget a friend to test in every morning after meditation. It ought that will help you stay with it for an extended term.

Locate a community. Even higher, discover a set of individuals who meditate and be part of them. This might be a Zen or Tibetan community close to you, wherein you may meditate alongside them. Alternatively, be part of an internet network and take a look at in with them to ask questions, advantage assist, and encourage others. My Sea Change Programme has a comparable community.

When you're completed, smile. When you've completed your mins, grin. Be happy that you had this time to yourself, which you saved your phrase, that you tested your trustworthiness, and that you took the opportunity to get to realise and end up pals with yourself. That turned into an first rate mins of your lifestyles.

Meditation isn't continuously clean or quiet. However, it has in reality first rate advantages that you may begin nowadays and preserve for the relaxation of your life.

Chapter 14: Mindfulness for Teens

Mindfulness refers to giving your entire hobby to the prevailing 2d without judgment. Many sports activities can be completed mindfully, which consist of exercise, painting, coloring, and fishing. There are also unique mindfulness wearing sports activities and strategies which can be suitable for young adults, together with paced respiration, grounding and body scans.

What Is Mindfulness?

Mindfulness is the intentional act of giving your undivided attention to the present second (vs. The beyond or future) with out judgment. The nonjudgmental mind-set is pinnacle, due to the reality we normally generally tend to choose our non-public thoughts, and in fact being aware of our mind can carry a radical exchange. Mindfulness for children and teens may be a extraordinary approach to help useful resource in improvement and as a coping information for hard times.

Benefits of Practicing Mindfulness For Teens

Mindfulness can help humans emerge as more privy to their mind and feelings, and that progressed belief can open doors to new selections. A centerpiece of mindfulness is looking at the prevailing without judgment—studying to meet oneself without judgment can construct compassion and kindness.

In nowadays's worldwide of fast-transferring media, interest can be difficult. Many mindfulness sports activities encourage sustained recognition, that might help in developing this talent.

Research has installed the following benefits of mindfulness for teenagers:1,2,three,four,5,6,7

Increases optimism

Improves social behaviors

Improvements in hobby

Improves electricity of will

Reduces bullying

Decreases teenager stressors and teen anxiety

Improves compassion towards oneself

Improves emotion regulation

Improves college conduct

11 Mindful Activities for Teens

Mindfulness activities that resonate collectively together along with your goals can be finished on a every day foundation. It's OK to start being aware with the resource of trying some of strategies to peer which of them healthy. Different sports activities can also furthermore have precise benefits; a few also can encourage relaxation, on the equal time as others may additionally additionally encourage recognition. Mindfulness for teens may be physical, intellectual, emotional, or non secular.

Here are 11 conscious sports for teens:

1. Deep Breathing

Breathwork is a traditional mindfulness hobby, which normally refers to purposefully manipulating the breath while mindfully specializing in it. This unique interest refers to deep, sluggish breaths (now and again referred to as stomach breaths) that use the diaphragm. This encourages your frame to loosen up.

2. Paced Breathing

An greater form of breath paintings is paced breathing, in which the period of the inhales and exhales are purposefully manipulated. It can be useful to have an prolonged exhale than inhale, because our coronary coronary coronary heart rate barely slows in some unspecified time in the future of the exhale. Try breathing in to a depend of 5, and exhaling to a count number number of 7. Use the competencies from the preceding sports (deep breathing) so your breaths are diaphragmatic.

3. Progressive Muscle Relaxation

Progressive muscle rest refers to tensing and releasing unique muscle organizations. For instance, scrunch your shoulders up in your ears; deliver as masses anxiety as viable in your neck and shoulders. Slowly matter to three and release all that tension. Now keep that with all muscle groups, collectively together with your hands, arms, chest, and stomach. You can do large or smaller muscle businesses relying in your options.

four. Meditation

There are many kinds of meditation, which generally contain maintaining one physical characteristic and paying attention to one hassle, like your respiration, a mantra, or bodily sensations. When your thoughts wanders—and it'll—nonjudgmentally supply it lower back to that issue of hobby. Meditating may be uncomfortable in the starting, and may not be suitable for a long term. If it feels too uncomfortable, it's OK to use exceptional mindfulness sports activities.

five. Grounding With 5-4-three-2-1

The five-four-3-2-1 exercise brings young adults, or people of any age, over again to the triumphing second via all of their senses.

Notice and say out loud or internally:

5 subjects you can see (pick a colour, for example, five blue topics)

four sensations you can feel (e.G., your decrease lower back in competition to the chair, cool air for your arms)

3 sounds you may pay interest

2 matters you may heady scent (it's OK to actively scent topics, just like the laundry detergent for your garments)

1 element you could taste

6. Body Scan

Completing a frame test is each other clean mindfulness interest. Bring your hobby to various additives of your frame, perhaps spending 10-30 seconds on each part (e.G., feet, bottoms of ft, tops of toes). Notice any and all bodily sensations: warmth, coolness, anxiety, tingling, strain, ache, or textures. There are many guided frame scans to assist facilitate this as properly.

7. Journaling

Journaling can definitely bear in thoughts, mainly while it's miles given complete interest with out judgment. Journaling can be achieved as a "loose write," in that you write some issue consists of mind without improving or censoring. Prompts additionally may be used to guide the writing in the direction of particular topics.

eight. Movement/Exercise

The repetitive movements of exercise can turn out to be meditative even as given one's complete hobby. Really any physical interest can turn out to be a mindfulness interest when approached with the thoughts-set of mindfulness. Take a aware walk and word the whole lot round you: sounds, the temperature, the way it feels to walk, physical sensations, nature, and points of hobby of the location.

nine. Coloring

An approachable mindfulness hobby is coloring. Coloring can convey a feel of creativity and playfulness to mindfulness. To make this a conscious interest, provide your entire attention to the coloring. When the mind wanders, lightly and nonjudgmentally deliver it once more to the coloring.

10. Listen to Music

Listen to a favorite tune together with your entire hobby. You can near their eyes and take note of everything. You want to try and notice how the tune makes you feel as well.

eleven. Mindful Eating

For a bit-sized mindfulness interest, strive consuming a chunk of fruit or a candy mindfully. Use a clementine as a start line; phrase the colour and texture of the fruit;

peel it slowly; take a look at the scent. Take one chunk and slowly take a look at what it's need to consume it.

How to Stick to a Mindfulness Practice

Mindfulness is simplest even as it is practiced often. Sometimes it could sense like a whole lot of hard work to attach yourself to a current dependancy. To do this, you could want to understand the type of mindfulness which you revel in, and decide out a way to make it sustainable for yourself. As a beginner to mindfulness, this can suggest experimenting with one-of-a-type methods.

Here are eight procedures young adults can preserve up with mindfulness practices:

1. Find a few element you revel in: in case you enjoy the exercising itself, it's an awful lot less difficult to return to it. If one mindfulness activity does now not resonate, that is OK! Try every other and discover some issue you need.

2. Keep it attainable: if the mindfulness workout is simply too lengthy or hard, pare it down. It is OK if it's handiest 1, 2, or 5 minutes! While 20 minutes of meditation is tremendous, so is 5 mins of coloring constant with day. Start small and allow the mindfulness exercise to expand organically.

three. Pair it with an gift addiction: dependancy researchers have located that a dependancy may be reinforced thru pairing it with an modern-day-day dependancy. For example, if you sweep your enamel every morning, do your mindfulness proper after. Or in case you always have a observe earlier than bed, carry out a bit conscious respiration proper earlier than.Eight

four. Create a reward for the addiction: you may sincerely make more potent the dependancy through growing a few shape of praise.Eight The reward need to be motivating to you—perhaps you could use a dependancy-tracker app, in which you may take a look at off your successes. Maybe you need to get a Starbucks drink each time you complete your mindfulness dependancy.

five. Find the right time of day: some of us are morning humans, and some of us are night owls. This is great! Use this data to finish your mindfulness interest at the time of the day in which your energy is right. For instance, in case you're too tired inside the morning, don't do it then.

6. Find a friend: having some companionship and responsibility let you commit yourself to a mindfulness dependancy. Find someone to companion with to make it more amusing!

7. Create a menu for yourself: in case you are having a hard time sticking to the same addiction each day, try switching it up. Create a menu of mindfulness sports. It may be as short or so long as you'd like, but supply yourself permission to strive numerous things.

eight. Set up a reminder or alarm: use your telephone or a smart speaker to installation a reminder for the time you decided as an first-rate healthy for you.

Final Thoughts

Mindful sports activities can be a exceptional device to help teenagers control their feelings and the demanding, chaotic nature of their lives. Luckily, there are numerous equipment for mindfulness so that everybody can find some component this is appropriate for them.

Epilogue

As we method the pinnacle of our highbrow exploration within the "Beginners Guide To Guided Meditation," I desire to express my sincere appreciation to you, esteemed reader, for becoming a member people in this profound and lifestyles-changing adventure. Throughout this discourse, we have explored the intellectual terrain, manoeuvred through the fluctuations of respiratory, and touched upon the profundities of inner tranquilly.

Beyond mere facts dissemination, the reason of this guide comes to be to ignite a profound transformation for your notion of yourself and the surrounding international. Guided meditation is not a set endpoint, however as an opportunity an ongoing way—a journey that transcends the confines of those pages and into the fabric of your ordinary life.

Remember, as you reflect at the practices located and the insights obtained, that the essence of meditation is the purpose to be gift, not perfection. One might also moreover possibly find out the profound insights of mindfulness at some level inside the ones times of tranquilly amidst the dynamic nature of life.

The epilogue features as a souvenir—a diffused prod to similarly expand the essence of meditation. Utilise it as an impetus for positive transformation, a wellspring of resilience for the duration of difficult intervals, and a compass that directs you in the direction of your inner sanctuary.

May the reverberations of your aware voyage resonate in some unspecified time inside the future of the terrific symphony of existence, producing vibrations of tranquilly and concord in every your personal lifestyles and the lives of these for your area. The practices you've cultivated aren't constrained to the pages of this manual; they'll be seeds planted within the fertile soil of your consciousness, organized to flourish inside the lawn of your reviews.

As you end this economic disaster, recognize that the journey of self-discovery is endless, and each breath is an opportunity to reconnect with the winning 2nd. Carry the commands discovered out proper right here as beacons of moderate, illuminating the course to a extra conscious and satisfying life.

Chapter 15: Understanding Stress

1. Definition and Types of Stress:

Before we embark on the adventure of relaxation and pressure cut charge, it's far essential to realize the very essence of strain. Stress is a herbal response to demanding conditions or dreams, a organic mechanism designed to mobilize our belongings for motion. However, the contemporary international regularly bombards us with stressors that surpass the adaptive capacities of this mechanism.

In this economic catastrophe, we will delve into the multifaceted nature of strain, exploring acute strain introduced approximately with the useful resource of on the spot stressful situations and chronic stress that lingers over extended intervals. By information the sorts of pressure, you benefit perception into the numerous strategies it may arise for your existence.

2. The Impact of Chronic Stress on Physical and Mental Health:

Chronic stress, whilst left unchecked, will become extra than a fleeting pain; it evolves right proper into a silent disruptor of our nicely-being. The non-stop activation of the frame's stress response device can reason a cascade of damaging results on each physical and highbrow fitness.

We'll discover how continual stress contributes to conditions which include cardiovascular problems, compromised immune function, and heightened dangers of highbrow fitness problems. Understanding the profound effect on our commonplace fitness is step one towards understanding the vital want for powerful pressure control techniques.

three. Common Symptoms of Stress:

Stress is not generally without problems recognizable; its signs and symptoms can display up in severa strategies, affecting everything of our lives. In this segment, we're able to light up the common signs and symptoms and signs and symptoms and signs that stress may be silently infiltrating your each day revel in. Whether it is physical manifestations like headaches and muscle anxiety or cognitive symptoms and symptoms which consist of trouble concentrating and irritability, spotting the ones signs empowers you to address strain at its roots.

By comprehending the definition, kinds, and signs and symptoms of pressure, you lay the foundation for a greater profound facts of your personal reports. As we maintain our exploration, you may discover how guided meditation becomes a incredible best friend in navigating and assuaging the burdens of strain, leading you towards a direction of tranquility and nicely-being.

Benefits of Guided Meditation

1. Overview of the Science behind Meditation and Stress Reduction:

Guided meditation isn't clearly a subjective exercising; its miles grounded in a wealthy tapestry of medical records. In this financial disaster, we can discover the fascinating era in the back of meditation and its profound effect on stress discount. From adjustments in brainwave patterns to the modulation of stress hormones, you will advantage insights into the complicated strategies wherein guided meditation influences our neurobiology.

Understanding the generation behind meditation offers a strong foundation, dispelling any skepticism and reinforcing the legitimacy of guided meditation as a effective device for pressure manipulate. As we resolve the mysteries of the mind-body connection, you'll recognize the transformative capability that lies in the smooth act of guided meditation.

2. Emotional, Mental, and Physical Benefits:

The blessings of guided meditation growth an extended way beyond the tranquility experienced inside the direction of a consultation. This section explores the holistic spectrum of blessings, beginning from emotional well-being to highbrow readability and physical fitness. We'll delve into how guided meditation acts as a catalyst for emotional regulation, stress resilience, greater suitable attention, or maybe tangible improvements in bodily health markers.

By the end of this economic catastrophe, you will have a whole understanding of the multifaceted benefits that guided meditation can deliver to your lifestyles. It's now not quite plenty calming the thoughts; it's far approximately fostering a country of well-being that permeates every detail of your life.

3. Real-existence Examples or Case Studies Illustrating Positive Outcomes:

The evidence of the pudding is inside the consuming, and the identical holds actual for guided meditation. In this segment, we are going to carry the advantages to life through real-lifestyles examples and case research. These narratives will show off how people, handling numerous disturbing conditions and stressors, have skilled tangible enhancements in their lives through the steady exercise of guided meditation.

Whether it's far overcoming chronic anxiety, improving sleep best, or carrying out a heightened experience of inner peace, the ones recollections will serve as beacons of concept, demonstrating that the benefits of guided meditation are not theoretical but transformative within the real worldwide.

As we discover those profound advantages, you'll be organized with the information and motivation to absolutely encompass guided meditation as a cornerstone of your adventure closer to rest and strain discount.

Chapter 16: Guided Meditation

1. Creating a Conducive Environment for Meditation:

Embarking at the direction of guided meditation calls for a place that nurtures serenity and awareness In this segment, we're going to explore a way to carve out a tranquil sanctuary within the midst of our bustling lives. From choosing the right physical space to incorporating factors like easy lighting and soothing sounds, you can discover ways to create an environment conducive to deepening your meditation workout.

Understanding how your environment has an impact to your mental kingdom is a pivotal first step. Whether it's far a committed meditation nook in your private home or locating solace in nature, the right surroundings can appreciably beautify the effectiveness of guided meditation.

2. Proper Posture and Breathing Techniques:

The body is both the anchor and the vessel inside the exercise of guided meditation. This segment delves into the significance of adopting a proper posture to facilitate relaxation and recognition. From seated positions to the feature of spinal alignment, you may discover how the physical detail of meditation intertwines with its highbrow and emotional dimensions.

Breathing serves due to the fact the gateway to a centered kingdom of thoughts. We'll explore diverse breathing techniques that complement guided meditation, improving your capability to calm the mind and sell a experience of presence. As you hold close the paintings of posture and breath, you may discover a harmonious synergy among your body and the guided meditation enjoy.

3. Addressing Common Misconceptions or Concerns approximately Meditation:

Meditation, on the identical time as widely stated for its advantages, is not evidence in opposition to misconceptions. In this a part of the monetary spoil, we can debunk not unusual myths and deal with issues that can act as boundaries to starting or maintaining a meditation exercising. Whether it's far the notion that one should clean the thoughts completely or the misconception that meditation is solely for non secular pastimes, we will offer clarity to empower you to your meditation adventure.

By dispelling those misconceptions, you could technique guided meditation with a refreshed perspective, unfastened from useless constraints. As we navigate through the sensible elements of making an environment, perfecting posture, and dispelling myths, you may be nicely-prepared to encompass the transformative potential of guided meditation with self guarantee and simplicity.

Types of Guided Meditations

1. Body Scan Meditation:

Embark on a adventure of self-discovery as we discover the profound workout of frame test meditation. This approach entails directing targeted hobby to top notch factors of the body, fostering a heightened cognizance of bodily sensations. Learn how the frame take a look at meditation may be a powerful tool for releasing tension and promoting relaxation from head to toe.

2. Mindfulness Meditation:

Dive into the essence of the present second with mindfulness meditation. This timeless exercising involves cultivating an recognition of mind, emotions, and sensations without judgment. Discover how mindfulness meditation complements your capability to stay grounded in the now, fostering intellectual readability and emotional balance.

3. Loving-Kindness Meditation:

Open your coronary coronary heart to the transformative power of loving-kindness meditation. This exercising involves directing benevolent thoughts and goals within the route of oneself and others. Explore how cultivating emotions of love and compassion can't handiest reduce pressure but furthermore deepen your connections with those spherical you.

4. Visualization Meditation:

Unlock the progressive ability of your mind through visualization meditation. This approach harnesses the electricity of creativeness, guiding you through intellectual photos and scenes that evoke relaxation and positivity. Delve into the arena of visualization meditation and discover how it is able to be a gateway to internal peace and pressure bargain.

5. Breathing Meditation:

Return to the critical rhythm of life with breathing meditation. Explore severa respiration techniques that feature anchors on your meditation exercise. Learn how conscious, intentional breathing may be a gateway to rest, helping to calm the thoughts and alleviate stress.

6. Mantra Meditation:

Immerse your self inside the rhythmic cadence of mantra meditation. This exercising includes repeating a word, word, or sound, imparting a focal point in your meditation. Uncover the soothing and centering consequences of mantra meditation, promoting a sense of tranquility and intellectual stillness.

7. Walking Meditation:

Embrace movement as a pathway to mindfulness with strolling meditation. Discover how the easy act of taking walks may be converted right into a meditative workout, fostering a harmonious connection among body and mind. Learn strategies to supply mindfulness to each step, selling rest and strain bargain through movement.

As we discover those various varieties of guided meditations, you may have the possibility to locate the approach that resonates maximum with you. Each approach gives a completely precise access difficulty to

Rest and pressure good buy, allowing you to tailor your meditation workout to suit your options and dreams.

Chapter 17: Designing Your Guided Meditation Sessions

1. Planning the Duration and Frequency of Sessions:

Embarking on a guided meditation adventure calls for considerate attention of time and frequency. In this section, we can find out the surest duration for meditation instructions and the manner regularly you need to have interaction on this practice. Whether you have were given have been given a few minutes or a extra extended length, find out the manner to tailor your meditation lessons to align with your life-style on the identical time as maximizing the advantages of relaxation and pressure discount.

2. Crafting Effective Scripts for Different Types of Meditations:

The coronary coronary coronary heart of guided meditation lies inside the carefully crafted scripts that manual your highbrow adventure. We'll delve into the paintings of script creation, exploring techniques for crafting powerful and resonant narratives for diverse meditation types. From frame check meditations to loving-kindness practices, discover ways to weave phrases that foster a experience of calm, mindfulness, and inner exploration.

3. Incorporating Background Music or Nature Sounds:

Enhance the sensory enjoy of guided meditation via exploring the location of records song or nature sounds. Discover how the proper auditory elements can complement one-of-a-kind meditation practices, growing an immersive and soothing surroundings. Whether it's miles the slight rustling of leaves or calming instrumental tunes, we're able to manual you in choosing and incorporating audio elements that increase the effectiveness of your meditation training.

As we navigate thru the intricacies of designing your guided meditation durations, you may gain insights into how each element contributes to a holistic and tailor-made revel in. By the forestall of this financial wreck, you may be geared up with the equipment to curate durations that seamlessly combine into your recurring, supplying a sanctuary of tranquility amid the dreams of each day life.

Overcoming Challenges

1. Dealing with Distractions during Meditation:

Distractions are inevitable partners on the journey of meditation. In this chapter, we are going to discover sensible techniques to navigate and decrease distractions, whether or no longer they get up from out of doors resources or internal mind. From establishing a devoted region to the usage of mindfulness strategies, learn how to cultivate attention and serenity amid the inevitable noise of the outside worldwide and the chatter inside.

2. Managing Expectations and Patience:

Patience isn't best a distinctive feature; it's miles a cornerstone of a satisfying meditation workout. We'll delve into the significance of managing expectancies, knowledge that meditation is a capacity that develops over the years. Discover strategies to encompass the ebb and go with the flow of your meditation research, fostering a mindset of persistence and self-compassion. By recalibrating your expectations, you may open the door to a extra sustainable and profitable meditation journey.

three. Addressing Common Obstacles to Consistent Practice:

Consistency is the crucial component to unlocking the general functionality of guided meditation. This section addresses commonplace obstacles that may prevent a ordinary exercising, which includes time constraints, motivation dips, or emotions of restlessness. Explore actionable techniques to conquer those hurdles, turning demanding situations into possibilities for increase and resilience. By cultivating a thoughts-set of adaptability and perseverance, you could assemble a basis for a sustainable and enduring meditation workout.

As we navigate through the nuances of overcoming demanding situations in guided meditation, you will emerge with a toolbox of practical strategies and a renewed experience of resilience. By embracing distractions, handling expectations, and addressing obstacles head-on, you may make more potent your dedication to rest and pressure discount thru the transformative energy of guided meditation.

Integrating Meditation into Daily Life

1. Incorporating Short Meditation Sessions into a Busy Schedule:

For many, the idea of meditation conjures pictures of lengthy intervals in serene environments. However, on this bankruptcy, we're going to find out the electricity of brief yet impactful meditation moments which can seamlessly combine into even the busiest schedules. Discover practical techniques for incorporating brief, targeted meditation classes for the duration of your day, permitting you to harness the benefits of rest and strain reduce charge without disrupting the go with the flow of your every day existence.

2. Using Meditation for Specific Situations (Work Stress, Family Challenges, and so forth.):

Meditation is a flexible tool that can be customized to address precise stressful situations. Explore the way to tailor your meditation exercise to navigate the intricacies of every day life, from place of work pressure to own family worrying situations. We'll delve into targeted meditation strategies that empower you to find out calm and clarity within the midst of particular situations, fostering resilience and emotional well-being.

3. Tips for Maintaining a Long-Term Meditation Practice:

Consistency is the linchpin of a a achievement meditation workout. This section offers realistic tips and techniques that will help you keep your commitment to guided meditation over the long term. From putting practical desires to establishing duty measures, you can learn how to domesticate a addiction that becomes an essential a part of your day by day normal. Discover the delight and success that comes from weaving meditation seamlessly into the material of your existence.

As we discover those techniques for integrating meditation into every day life, you may discover that the transformative strength of guided meditation extends a long way beyond dedicated periods. It turns into a dynamic and adaptable tool, empowering you to navigate the challenges of normal lifestyles with greater ease, resilience, and a sense of internal peace.

Additional Resources

1. Recommended Books, Apps, and Websites for Guided Meditations:

Dive deeper into the arena of guided meditation with a curated preference of belongings. This phase gives guidelines for books, apps, and websites that provide a wealth of guided meditation training. From insightful reads to interactive applications and on line structures, you may discover loads of tools to enhance and diversify your meditation journey. Explore the services of experienced guides and authors to discover the property that resonate most together together with your selections and desires.

2. Information on Local Meditation Groups or Classes:

Community help can extensively growth your meditation experience. Uncover the advantages of connecting with like-minded people via the use of exploring community meditation groups or instructions. This phase offers steerage on locating and becoming a member of in-individual or virtual groups in which you could share opinions, gather steering, and foster a feel of camaraderie to your meditation course. Engaging with others can provide precious insights and encouragement as you continue to refine your exercise.

3. Suggestions for Further Reading and Research:

www.ingramcontent.com/pod-product-compliance
Lightning Source LLC
Chambersburg PA
CBHW072157070526
44585CB00015B/1183